INTRODUCTION

Welcome to a journey towards vibrant health, vitality, and well-being! In the cacophony of dietary trends and fads, the Ornish diet shines as a beacon of evidence-based wisdom and profound nourishment. This book is your comprehensive guide to unlocking the transformative power of the Ornish approach to nutrition, tailored specifically for the dynamic, health-conscious young adult.

As you embark on this journey, prepare to delve into the heart of holistic wellness, where food isn't merely fuel but a profound expression of self-care and compassion. Dr. Dean Ornish's groundbreaking research has illuminated the path towards reversing chronic diseases and embracing vitality through simple yet profound dietary choices. Whether you're seeking to kickstart your health journey or deepen your understanding of mindful nutrition, this book is your trusted companion.

CHAPTER ONE

The Ornish diet philosophy

The Ornish approach is more than just using food as fuel; it's about realising how closely our dietary decisions affect our physical health, emotional stability, spiritual harmony, and overall physical well-being.

Central to the Ornish philosophy is the recognition that our bodies are not isolated systems but intricately woven tapestries where every choice reverberates across multiple dimensions of our existence. This holistic perspective serves as the guiding principle behind the Ornish diet, inviting us to nurture not just our physical bodies but our entire being.

The Ornish diet is not merely a set of dietary guidelines but a way of life, an invitation to cultivate mindfulness and intentionality in our relationship with food. It encourages us to view food not just as sustenance but as medicine, recognising the profound impact it has on our health and well-being. By embracing whole, plant-based foods rich in nutrients and antioxidants, we nourish our bodies at a cellular level, fostering vitality and resilience.

The Science Behind The Ornish Approach

The cornerstone of the Ornish approach lies in its ability to reverse chronic diseases—a feat once deemed improbable, if not impossible, by conventional medical wisdom. Yet, through meticulous research and clinical practice, the Ornish method has emerged as a beacon of hope for millions grappling with conditions such as heart disease, diabetes, and hypertension.

At the forefront of this paradigm shift is the transformative power of plant-based nutrition. Decades of research have elucidated the myriad benefits of a diet rich in fruits, vegetables, whole grains, and legumes—a veritable cornucopia of micronutrients and phytochemicals that exert a profound influence on our health. By embracing plant-based foods and minimising the consumption of animal products and processed foods, individuals can mitigate inflammation, improve endothelial function, and enhance cardiovascular health— a testament to the potent healing properties of nature's bounty.

Central to the Ornish approach is the concept of lifestyle medicine—a holistic framework that recognises the pivotal role of lifestyle factors in the prevention and treatment of chronic diseases. Through a synergistic blend of dietary modifications, regular physical activity, stress management techniques, and social support, individuals can address the root causes of illness and foster a state of vibrant well-being. From the tranquil shores of mindfulness meditation to the invigorating rhythms of cardiovascular exercise, each facet of the Ornish lifestyle serves as a potent elixir for body, mind, and spirit.

Crucially, the Ornish approach extends beyond the realm of disease management to embrace the transformative potential of community and connection. Through the support of like-minded individuals and the guidance of trained professionals, individuals embarking on the Ornish journey find themselves enveloped in a web of support and encouragement—a nurturing environment where healing flourishes and hope blossoms.

The scientific evidence supporting the Ornish approach is nothing short of compelling. Landmark studies have demonstrated not only the reversal of coronary artery disease but also improvements in insulin sensitivity, blood pressure, and cholesterol levels—a testament to the profound impact of lifestyle interventions on our physiological well-being. Moreover, emerging research suggests that the benefits of the Ornish approach extend far beyond the realm of cardiovascular health, encompassing a diverse array of conditions ranging from cancer to autoimmune disorders—a testament to the universality of its principles and the resilience of the human spirit.

Exploring The Four Key Pillars

These pillars—plant-based nutrition, exercise, stress management, and social support—serve as cornerstones of a holistic lifestyle that fosters vitality, resilience, and inner harmony. Let us embark on a journey of exploration, unravelling the mysteries of each pillar and discovering their profound impact on our lives.

Plant-Based Nutrition:

At the heart of the Ornish approach lies the transformative power of plant-based nutrition. By centering our diets around fruits, vegetables, whole grains, and legumes, we harness the healing energy of nature's bounty, nourishing our bodies at a cellular level. Plant-based foods are not merely sources of sustenance but repositories of life-giving nutrients—vitamins, minerals, antioxidants, and phytochemicals—that fortify our bodies against disease and dysfunction. From the vibrant hues of leafy greens to the rich flavours of ripe berries, each bite offers a symphony of taste and nourishment—a testament to the abundance of nature's bounty and the wisdom of choosing foods that honour our bodies and the planet.

Exercise:

Regular physical activity is a cornerstone of the Ornish lifestyle, offering a myriad of benefits for the body, mind, and spirit. Whether it's brisk walking, yoga, or strength training, exercise serves as a potent elixir for cardiovascular health, muscular strength, and emotional well-being. Through movement, we cultivate vitality and resilience, invigorating our bodies with the life force of motion. Moreover, exercise is a powerful antidote to stress, anxiety, and depression, offering a sanctuary of solace and rejuvenation in an increasingly hectic world. By integrating regular physical activity into our daily lives, we embrace the joy of movement and the profound sense of aliveness it brings.

Stress Management:

In today's fast-paced world, stress has emerged as a ubiquitous companion—a silent assailant that erodes our health and diminishes our vitality. Yet, in the face of adversity, we possess the power to cultivate inner peace and resilience through the practice of stress management techniques. Whether it's mindfulness meditation, deep breathing exercises, or progressive muscle relaxation, these tools offer a sanctuary of serenity amidst the chaos of modern life. By cultivating awareness and presence, we untangle the knots of stress that bind us, reclaiming our inner equilibrium and restoring balance to body, mind, and spirit.

Social Support:

Human beings are inherently social creatures, wired for connection and community. In the Ornish approach, social support serves as a vital pillar of well-being, offering a lifeline of encouragement, empathy, and camaraderie in times of need. Whether it's the embrace of family, the laughter of friends, or the guidance of support groups, social connections nourish our souls and uplift our spirits. Through the bonds of fellowship, we find solace in shared experiences and strength in unity, navigating life's challenges with grace and resilience.

The Power Of Plants

From the lush greens of spinach to the vibrant hues of bell peppers, the bounty of the earth offers a symphony of flavours, textures, and nutrients that nourish not only our bodies but also our souls. Let us embark on a journey of exploration, unravelling the mysteries of plant-powered nutrition and discovering its profound impact on our health and well-being.

The Abundance of Nature:

At the heart of plant-powered nutrition lies the boundless abundance of nature's pantry—a treasure trove of fruits, vegetables, whole grains, and legumes that offer a cornucopia of vitamins, minerals, antioxidants, and phytonutrients. From the crisp sweetness of apples to the creamy richness of avocados, each plant-based food offers a unique array of nutrients that fortify our bodies against disease and dysfunction. By embracing the diversity of plant foods, we nourish ourselves at a cellular level, fostering vitality and resilience from the inside out.

Harnessing the Healing Power of Plants:

Plants are not merely sources of sustenance but repositories of healing energy—a potent elixir that offers relief from the ailments that afflict us. Decades of research have elucidated the myriad benefits of a plant-based diet, from reducing inflammation and improving cardiovascular health to enhancing immune function and promoting longevity. By centering our diets around plant-powered foods, we harness the innate healing wisdom of nature, reclaiming our health and vitality with each nourishing bite.

The Wisdom of Whole Foods:

In the age of processed foods and convenience cuisine, the wisdom of whole foods shines brightly as a beacon of health and vitality. Whole, unprocessed plant foods offer a symphony of nutrients in their natural form, free from the additives, preservatives, and artificial ingredients that pervade our modern food supply. By choosing whole foods over processed counterparts, we honor the innate intelligence of nature, embracing foods that nourish our bodies and uplift our spirits with their purity and vitality.

Cultivating Connection:

In embracing plant-powered nutrition, we cultivate a

profound connection—not only with our bodies but with the earth itself. By choosing foods that honour the planet and its inhabitants, we participate in a sacred act of reciprocity, fostering harmony and balance in our relationship with the natural world. Moreover, plant-powered nutrition offers a pathway to connection with others as we share meals, recipes, and culinary traditions that celebrate the abundance of the earth and the joy of nourishing ourselves and each other.

Building A Colorful Plate

Let us explore the vibrant tapestry of flavours, textures, and nutrients that these foods offer, enriching our diets and nourishing our bodies and souls in equal measure.

The Rainbow of Nutrients:

When it comes to building a colourful plate, diversity is key. Each colour in the plant kingdom corresponds to a unique array of nutrients, each essential for vibrant health and well-being. From the deep purples of blueberries, rich in antioxidants, to the fiery oranges of sweet potatoes, packed with beta-carotene, every hue offers a symphony of vitamins, minerals, and phytonutrients that fortify our bodies and protect against disease. By embracing the rainbow of plant-based foods, we ensure that our plates are not only visually stunning but nutritionally complete, offering a bounty of health-promoting compounds with each delicious bite.

Fruits:

Fruits are nature's sweet gift, offering a tantalising blend of sweetness and nutrition. Whether it's the juicy crunch of apples, the succulent flesh of mangoes, or the tart tang of strawberries, fruits offer a diverse array of flavours and textures that awaken the senses and delight the palate. Rich in vitamins, minerals, and antioxidants, fruits nourish our bodies with their natural goodness, offering a guilt-free indulgence that satisfies both hunger and cravings.

Vegetables:

Vegetables are the unsung heroes of the plant kingdom, offering a wealth of nutrients in a low-calorie package. From the crisp crunch of bell peppers to the earthy sweetness of carrots, vegetables offer a kaleidoscope of flavours and textures that elevate any meal from ordinary to extraordinary. Packed with vitamins, minerals, and fibre, vegetables support our health and vitality with their nutritional bounty, promoting optimal digestion, immune function, and cellular health.

Whole Grains:

Whole grains are the backbone of a healthy diet, offering sustained energy and satiety with their complex carbohydrates and fiber. Whether it's the nutty richness of quinoa, the chewy texture of brown rice, or the hearty goodness of oats, whole grains provide a versatile canvas upon which to build nutritious and satisfying meals. Rich in vitamins, minerals, and antioxidants, whole grains offer a myriad of health benefits, from promoting heart health and weight management to regulating blood sugar levels and enhancing digestion.

Legumes:

Legumes are nutritional powerhouses, offering a potent blend of protein, fibre, and essential nutrients. Whether it's the creamy comfort of lentils, the meaty texture of chickpeas, or the buttery goodness of edamame, legumes provide a versatile and delicious source of plant-based protein that supports muscle growth, repair, and maintenance. Rich in vitamins, minerals, and phytonutrients, legumes offer a host of health benefits, from lowering cholesterol and blood pressure to stabilising blood sugar levels and promoting digestive health.

Practical Tips For Incorporating Plant-Based Meals Into Your Lifestyle

Transitioning to a plant-based diet can feel like a daunting task, especially in a world inundated with convenience foods and meat-centric meals. Yet, with a bit of creativity, intentionality, and planning, incorporating more plant-based meals into your lifestyle can be both delicious and rewarding. Let us explore some practical tips to help you embark on this journey of nourishment and vitality, one plant-powered meal at a time.

Start Slowly:

For many people, the thought of giving up animal products entirely can be overwhelming. Instead of diving in headfirst, consider starting slowly by incorporating more plant-based meals into your routine gradually. Begin by replacing one or two meat-based meals per week with plant-based alternatives, such as veggie stir-fries, bean chilli, or lentil soup. As you become more comfortable with plant-based cooking and discover new recipes, you can gradually increase the number of plant-based meals in your repertoire.

Experiment with new ingredients:

One of the joys of plant-based cooking is the opportunity to experiment with a wide variety of fruits, vegetables, whole grains, and legumes. Don't be afraid to step outside of your culinary comfort zone and try new ingredients and flavour combinations. Visit your local farmers' market or grocery store and explore the seasonal produce section, selecting vibrant fruits and vegetables that catch your eye. Experiment with different cooking methods, such as roasting, steaming, sautéing, and grilling, to bring out the natural flavours and textures of plant-based ingredients.

Focus on Whole Foods:

When incorporating plant-based meals into your diet, focus on whole, unprocessed foods whenever possible. Choose whole grains such as quinoa, brown rice, and oats over refined grains like white rice and pasta. Opt for fresh or frozen fruits and vegetables instead of canned varieties, which may contain added sugars and preservatives. By prioritizing whole foods, you'll not only maximize the nutritional value of your meals but also enhance their flavor and satiety.

Get Creative with Flavour:

Plant-based cooking is anything but bland and boring. Experiment with herbs, spices, and condiments to add depth and complexity to your dishes. Incorporate fresh herbs like basil, cilantro, and mint into salads, soups, and sauces for a burst of flavor. Experiment with aromatic spices like cumin, turmeric, and paprika to elevate the taste of roasted vegetables, grains, and legumes. Explore ethnic cuisines such as Mediterranean, Asian, and Latin American, which are rich in plant-based ingredients and bold flavours.

Plan Ahead:

One of the keys to success with plant-based eating is planning ahead. Take some time each week to plan your meals and grocery list, taking into account your schedule, dietary preferences, and nutritional needs. Consider batch-cooking staple ingredients such as grains, beans, and roasted vegetables to have on hand for quick and easy meal assembly throughout the week. Invest in reusable storage containers to portion out meals and snacks for grab-and-go convenience.

The Art Of Mindful Eating

By cultivating mindful eating habits, we reconnect with the wisdom of our bodies, honouring the intricate dance of hunger, satiety, and satisfaction that guides us on our journey of health and well-being. Let us explore the art of mindful eating and discover its profound impact on our relationship with food and ourselves.

Presence and Awareness:

At its core, mindful eating is about presence and awareness—bringing our full attention to the sensory experience of eating with curiosity and non-judgement. Instead of mindlessly consuming food while distracted by screens, thoughts, or emotions, we invite ourselves to be fully present with each bite, engaging all of our senses to fully appreciate the flavours, textures, and aromas of the food before us. By cultivating this heightened awareness, we tap into the innate wisdom of our bodies, allowing hunger and satiety cues to guide our eating patterns in harmony with our physiological needs.

Savoring Each Bite:

Mindful eating is not just about what we eat but also how we eat it. It's about savouring each bite with intention and appreciation, allowing ourselves to fully experience the pleasure and nourishment that food has to offer. Whether it's the crisp crunch of an apple, the creamy richness of avocado, or the savoury aroma of a freshly cooked meal, each bite becomes a moment of mindfulness—a chance to pause, breathe, and connect with the present moment. By savoring each bite, we cultivate a deeper appreciation for the food we eat and the process of nourishing our bodies, fostering a sense of gratitude and reverence for the abundance of nature's bounty.

Honouring Hunger and Fullness

Mindful eating encourages us to listen to our bodies' innate signals of hunger and fullness, honouring the wisdom of our internal cues rather than external rules or restrictions. Instead of eating according to rigid schedules or arbitrary portion sizes, we tune in to the subtle sensations of hunger and satiety that arise within us, eating when we're hungry and stopping when we're comfortably satisfied. By attuning ourselves to these cues, we forge a deeper connection with our bodies and build trust in our ability to nourish ourselves in a way that feels satisfying and sustainable.

Cultivating Gratitude and Compassion:

Mindful eating is not just a practice of nourishing our bodies but also of nurturing our hearts and souls. It invites us to cultivate gratitude for the food we eat and the countless hands that brought it to our plates—from the farmers who grew it to the cooks who prepared it. By recognising the interconnectedness of all beings and the web of relationships that sustain us, we foster a sense of compassion and interconnectedness that extends beyond the boundaries of our own lives.

Overcoming Emotional Eating And Developing A Healthy Relationship With Food

We will explore the practice of mindful eating as a powerful tool for overcoming emotional eating and cultivating a healthier relationship with food.

Understanding Emotional Eating:

Emotional eating is a complex phenomenon rooted in the interplay of psychological, physiological, and environmental factors. It often involves using food as a means of coping with difficult emotions such as stress, anxiety, sadness, or loneliness. In times of emotional distress, food can provide temporary relief and distraction, offering a momentary escape from uncomfortable feelings. However, this reliance on food to soothe emotional pain can lead to a cycle of guilt, shame, and overeating, further exacerbating the underlying emotional issues.

The Role of Mindful Eating:

Mindful eating offers a powerful antidote to emotional eating by inviting us to cultivate awareness and presence around our eating habits. Instead of turning to food as a reflexive response to emotions, mindful eating encourages us to pause and inquire into the underlying causes of our cravings and desires. By tuning into our bodies' hunger and fullness cues, we can begin to differentiate between physical hunger and emotional hunger, allowing us to respond to our needs with greater clarity and intention.

Exploring the Root Causes

To overcome emotional eating, it's essential to explore the root causes of our emotional triggers and cravings. This may involve examining past experiences, traumas, or belief systems that contribute to our relationship with food. By shining a light on the underlying emotional patterns and conditioning that drive our eating behaviours, we can begin to cultivate a greater sense of self-awareness and empowerment, allowing us to make more conscious choices around food.

Practicing Self-Compassion:

Developing a healthy relationship with food requires practicing self-compassion and self-care. Instead of harsh self-judgement or criticism when we experience emotional eating episodes, we can offer ourselves kindness and understanding. Recognising that emotional eating is a natural response to emotional distress can help us approach ourselves with greater gentleness and empathy, fostering a sense of acceptance and forgiveness that allows us to move forward with greater resilience and grace.

Building Alternative Coping Strategies:

In addition to mindfulness, it's important to build alternative coping strategies for dealing with difficult emotions that don't involve food. This may include practicing stress-relief techniques such as deep breathing, meditation, or yoga, engaging in creative outlets such as journaling or art, or seeking support from friends, family, or mental health professionals. By cultivating a toolkit of healthy coping strategies, we can develop resilience and resourcefulness in the face of emotional challenges, reducing our reliance on food as our sole means of comfort and support.

Mindful Meal Planning And Preparation

The kitchen is more than just a space for preparing meals—it's a sanctuary of creativity, nourishment, and connection. By approaching meal planning and preparation with mindfulness and intentionality, we can transform the act of cooking into a joyful and soul-nourishing experience. In this chapter, we will explore the art of mindful meal planning and preparation, uncovering the secrets to fostering joy in the kitchen and cultivating a deeper connection with the food we eat.

Setting the stage:

Mindful meal planning begins long before we step foot in the kitchen—it starts with setting the stage for success. Take some time each week to plan your meals and create a shopping list, taking into account your dietary preferences, nutritional needs, and schedule. Consider incorporating a diverse array of fruits, vegetables, whole grains, and legumes into your meals to ensure a balance of nutrients and flavors. By approaching meal planning with intentionality, you set yourself up for success and create a foundation for nourishing and satisfying meals throughout the week.

Creating a Sacred Space:

The kitchen is a sacred space—a place where we come to nourish our bodies and feed our souls. Cultivate a sense of reverence and mindfulness as you enter the kitchen, treating each ingredient with care and respect. Take a moment to clear clutter from your countertops, light a candle, or play soft music to create a soothing atmosphere that invites presence and focus. By infusing your kitchen with intentionality and mindfulness, you create a space where cooking becomes a meditative practice—a chance to slow down, tune in, and savour the process of nourishing yourself and your loved ones.

Engaging the senses:

Cooking is a sensory experience—a symphony of sights, sounds, smells, tastes, and textures that delight the senses and awaken the soul. As you prepare your meals, engage all of your senses to fully immerse yourself in the experience. Notice the vibrant colours of fresh produce, the tantalising aromas of herbs and spices, the rhythmic sounds of chopping and stirring, and the mouthwatering tastes and textures of your creations. By tuning into your senses, you deepen your connection with the food you're preparing and enhance the pleasure of the cooking process.

Cultivating Creativity:

Cooking is an art—an expression of creativity and innovation that knows no bounds. Embrace your inner chef and experiment with new ingredients, flavours, and techniques to infuse your meals with excitement and variety. Try incorporating seasonal produce, ethnic cuisines, or plant-based alternatives into your cooking repertoire to expand your culinary horizons and stimulate your palate. By approaching cooking with curiosity and openness, you unleash your creativity and infuse your meals with joy and vitality.

Practicing Gratitude:

In the midst of busy schedules and hectic lives, it's easy to take the act of cooking for granted. Pause for a moment to cultivate gratitude for the food before you—the nourishing ingredients, the hands that grew and harvested them, and the love and care that went into preparing them. Reflect on the journey that each ingredient has taken to arrive on your plate, from seed to harvest to table. By practicing gratitude, you infuse your meals with love and appreciation, transforming the act of eating into a sacred ritual of connection and abundance.

Incorporating Aerobic Exercise And Strength Training For Optimal Health

Movement is the language of the body—a symphony of strength, flexibility, and vitality that echoes through every fibre of our being. In this chapter, we will explore the importance of incorporating aerobic exercise and strength training into our daily routines to nurture our bodies and cultivate vibrant health and well-being.

The Power of Aerobic Exercise:

Aerobic exercise is a cornerstone of a healthy lifestyle, offering a multitude of benefits for both the body and the mind. From brisk walking and jogging to cycling and swimming, aerobic exercise strengthens the heart, improves cardiovascular health, and enhances lung function. Moreover, aerobic exercise boosts mood, reduces stress, and promotes mental clarity and focus, making it a powerful antidote to the pressures of modern life. By incorporating aerobic exercise into our daily routines, we nourish our bodies with the oxygen and vitality they need to thrive.

Strength Training for Resilience:

Strength training is another essential component of a well-rounded exercise regimen, offering a host of benefits for muscle strength, bone density, and functional fitness. By engaging in resistance exercises such as weightlifting, bodyweight exercises, or resistance band workouts, we stimulate muscle growth and development, improve balance and coordination, and reduce the risk of injury and falls. Moreover, strength training boosts metabolism, promotes fat loss, and enhances overall physical performance, allowing us to move through life with grace, power, and resilience.

Balancing Cardiovascular and Strength Workouts:

Achieving optimal health and fitness requires a balanced approach that incorporates both aerobic exercise and strength training into our workout routines. Aim for a mix of cardiovascular workouts and strength training sessions throughout the week to maximise the benefits of each modality. Consider alternating days of aerobic exercise with days of strength training, allowing your body time to recover and adapt to the demands of each type of exercise. By striking a balance between cardiovascular and strength workouts, you create a comprehensive exercise programme that fosters health, vitality, and longevity.

Finding Joy in Movement:

Exercise is not just about building strength or burning calories; it's about finding joy in movement and celebrating the capabilities of our bodies. Explore different forms of exercise and physical activity to discover what brings you pleasure and fulfillment. Whether it's dancing, hiking, practicing yoga, or playing sports, find activities that resonate with your interests and passions, and make movement a source of joy and self-expression. By embracing movement as a celebration of life, you infuse your workouts with enthusiasm and vitality, fostering a lifelong commitment to health and well-being.

Listening to Your Body:

Above all, listen to your body and honour its wisdom. Pay attention to how you feel during and after exercise, and adjust your workouts accordingly. If you're feeling fatigued or sore, give yourself permission to rest and recover. If you're feeling energised and invigorated, seize the opportunity to challenge yourself and push your limits. By tuning into your body's signals and responding with kindness and compassion, you cultivate a deeper connection with yourself and lay the foundation for a lifetime of health and vitality.

Making movement a priority:

Incorporating aerobic exercise and strength training into your daily life requires commitment and consistency. Make movement a non-negotiable part of your routine by scheduling regular workouts and prioritising physical activity in your daily schedule. Find ways to integrate movement into your day-to-day life, whether it's taking the stairs instead of the elevator, walking or cycling to work, or scheduling active outings with friends and family. By making movement a priority, you invest in your health and well-being and set yourself up for a lifetime of vitality and longevity.

Finding Balance And Pleasure In Physical

Activity

Physical activity is not just about burning calories or building muscles—it's about finding joy, balance, and pleasure in movement. In this chapter, we will explore the importance of embracing a holistic approach to physical activity that honours the needs and desires of our bodies, fosters a sense of enjoyment and fulfilment, and promotes long-term health and well-being.

Honouring Your Body's Wisdom:

Our bodies are wise guides, speaking to us through sensations, feelings, and instincts. Listen to your body and honour its cues, recognising that movement should feel good and nourishing, not punishing or depleting. Pay attention to how different forms of physical activity make you feel—whether it's the exhilaration of a brisk walk, the serenity of yoga, or the invigoration of a dance class. Trust your intuition and choose activities that resonate with your body and soul, honouring the unique needs and preferences of your own being.

Embracing Variety and Versatility:

Variety is the spice of life, especially when it comes to physical activity. Explore a diverse range of activities and exercises to keep your workouts fresh, engaging, and enjoyable. Mix up your routine with activities that challenge different muscle groups, engage different energy systems, and stimulate different senses and emotions. Whether it's swimming, hiking, cycling, or practicing tai chi, embrace the versatility of movement and discover the infinite possibilities for joy and fulfilment that lie within.

Finding Flow and Presence:

Physical activity offers a gateway to presence—a state of flow where time seems to stand still and you become fully immersed in the moment. Cultivate mindfulness and presence in your workouts, focusing your attention on the sensations of your body, the rhythm of your breath, and the beauty of your surroundings. Let go of distractions and preoccupations, allowing yourself to be fully present with the experience of movement. By cultivating a sense of flow and presence in your physical activity, you tap into the transformative power of the present moment, fostering a deep sense of connection and aliveness.

Making Movement Playful and fun:

Physical activity doesn't have to be a chore—it can be playful, spontaneous, and downright fun. Rediscover the joy of movement by approaching exercise with a sense of curiosity and wonder, like a child exploring a new playground. Experiment with different movement modalities, inventing new games and challenges to keep your workouts engaging and exciting. Invite friends, family, or pets to join you in your adventures, turning exercise into a social activity that nourishes both body and soul. By infusing your workouts with playfulness and fun, you transform exercise from a task to be checked off a list into a source of pleasure and delight.

Honouring Rest and Recovery:

Rest and recovery are essential components of any balanced approach to physical activity. Listen to your body's signals of fatigue and exhaustion, and give yourself permission to rest and recharge when needed. Incorporate rest days into your workout schedule, allowing your body time to repair and rebuild after periods of exertion. Prioritise sleep, hydration, and nutrition to support your body's recovery process and ensure that you have the energy and vitality to continue enjoying movement for years to come.

Understanding The Impact Of Stress On Your Health

We will delve into the intricate relationship between stress and health, exploring how chronic stress impacts the body and mind, and discovering strategies for taming stress and cultivating resilience.

The Physiology of Stress:

When we encounter a stressful situation, whether it's a looming deadline at work or a heated argument with a loved one, our bodies initiate a cascade of physiological responses known as the stress response. This ancient survival mechanism, often referred to as the fight-or-flight response, triggers the release of stress hormones such as cortisol and adrenaline, preparing the body to react to perceived threats. While this response is essential for survival in the face of immediate danger, chronic activation of the stress response can have detrimental effects on our health over time.

The Impact on the Body:

Chronic stress takes a toll on virtually every system of the body, from the cardiovascular and immune systems to the digestive and nervous systems. Prolonged exposure to stress hormones can lead to a host of health problems, including high blood pressure, weakened immune function, digestive disorders, and an increased risk of chronic diseases such as heart disease, diabetes, and depression. Moreover, chronic stress can contribute to unhealthy coping mechanisms such as overeating, smoking, and substance abuse, further exacerbating the negative impact on health.

The Mind-Body Connection:

The relationship between stress and health is not limited to the physical body; it also extends to the realm of mental and emotional well-being. Chronic stress has been linked to an increased risk of anxiety, depression, and other mood disorders, as well as cognitive decline and impaired memory function. Moreover, stress can negatively impact our relationships, work performance, and overall quality of life, creating a vicious cycle of stress and dysfunction that can be difficult to break.

Strategies For Taming Stress

While stress is an inevitable part of life, there are steps we can take to mitigate its impact on our health and well-being. Cultivating mindfulness and awareness is a powerful tool for managing stress, allowing us to observe our thoughts, emotions, and bodily sensations with curiosity and non-judgement. By practicing mindfulness techniques such as deep breathing, meditation, and yoga, we can activate the body's relaxation response, counteracting the effects of the stress response and promoting a sense of calm and equilibrium.

Building Resilience:

In addition to managing stress in the moment, it's important to build resilience—the ability to bounce back from adversity and thrive in the face of challenges.

Cultivate resilience by fostering strong social connections, engaging in activities that bring you joy and fulfilment, and nurturing a sense of purpose and meaning in life. Develop healthy coping mechanisms for dealing with stress, such as exercise, creative expression, and spending time in nature. By building resilience, you empower yourself to navigate life's ups and downs with grace and fortitude, emerging stronger and more resilient with each passing challenge.

Harnessing The Power Of Relaxation Techniques And Meditation

Relaxation techniques and meditation offer powerful tools for taming stress, calming the mind, and cultivating resilience in the face of life's challenges. We will explore the transformative power of relaxation techniques and meditation, uncovering their profound effects on the body, mind, and spirit, and discovering practical strategies for incorporating them into our daily lives.

The Science of Relaxation:

Relaxation is not merely a luxury—it's a biological necessity for optimal health and well-being. When we engage in relaxation techniques such as deep breathing, progressive muscle relaxation, or guided imagery, we activate the body's relaxation response—a physiological state characterised by reduced heart rate, blood pressure, and muscle tension. This state of deep relaxation counteracts the effects of the stress response, promoting a sense of calm, balance, and rejuvenation throughout the body and mind.

The Benefits of Meditation:

Meditation is a powerful practice for quieting the mind, cultivating mindfulness, and enhancing resilience in the face of stress. By directing our attention inward and focusing on the present moment, meditation helps us develop greater awareness of our thoughts, emotions, and bodily sensations. Over time, regular meditation practice can rewire the brain, strengthening neural pathways associated with attention, emotional regulation, and stress resilience. Moreover, meditation has been shown to reduce symptoms of anxiety, depression, and other mood disorders and improve overall psychological well-being.

Practical Techniques for Relaxation and Meditation:

Incorporating relaxation techniques and meditation into your daily routine doesn't have to be complicated or time-consuming. Start by setting aside just a few minutes each day to practice deep breathing or progressive muscle relaxation. Find a quiet, comfortable space where you can sit or lie down without distractions, and close your eyes. Take slow, deep breaths, inhaling through your nose and exhaling through your mouth, focusing on the sensation of the breath moving in and out of your body. As you breathe, scan your body for areas of tension and consciously relax each muscle group, starting from your toes and working your way up to your head.

Cultivating Mindfulness Through Meditation:

Meditation is a practice of mindfulness—a state of open-hearted awareness and acceptance of the present moment. Begin with simple mindfulness meditation exercises, such as focused attention on the breath or body sensations. Sit quietly and observe your thoughts as they arise, without judgement or attachment, allowing them to come and go like clouds passing through the sky. If your mind wanders, gently guide your attention back to the present moment, anchoring yourself in the sensations of the breath or body. Over time, as you cultivate mindfulness through meditation, you'll develop greater clarity, resilience, and compassion towards yourself and others.

Integrating Relaxation and Meditation into Daily Life:

To reap the full benefits of relaxation techniques and meditation, integrate them into your daily life in meaningful and sustainable ways. Find moments throughout your day to pause and breathe, whether it's during your morning routine, on your lunch break, or before bed. Create a dedicated space in your home where you can practice meditation and relaxation without distractions, decorating it with items that inspire peace and tranquility. Consider joining a meditation group or attending mindfulness retreats to deepen your practice and connect with others on the path of self-discovery and growth.

Embracing the Journey:

Above all, remember that relaxation techniques and meditation are not about achieving a state of perfection or enlightenment—they're about embracing the journey of self-discovery and self-care. Approach your practice with openness and curiosity, allowing yourself to be present with whatever thoughts, emotions, or sensations arise. Cultivate a sense of gentleness and compassion towardss yourself as you navigate the ups and downs of life, trusting in the transformative power of relaxation and meditation to guide you towardss greater peace, resilience, and well-being.

Creating Balanced, Delicious Meals With Ease

By nourishing our bodies with wholesome, nutrient-rich foods, we lay the foundation for vitality, resilience, and longevity. We will explore practical tips and meal plans for creating balanced, delicious meals with ease, empowering you to take charge of your health and embrace the joy of nourishing yourself and your loved ones.

The Art of Balanced Nutrition:

Balanced nutrition is the cornerstone of a healthy diet, providing the essential nutrients our bodies need to thrive. A balanced meal typically consists of a variety of foods from all the major food groups, including fruits, vegetables, whole grains, lean proteins, and healthy fats. Aim to fill your plate with a rainbow of colourful fruits and vegetables, which are rich in vitamins, minerals, and antioxidants that support overall health and vitality. Incorporate whole grains such as brown rice, quinoa, and whole wheat pasta, which provide fibre and complex carbohydrates for sustained energy. Include lean proteins such as poultry, fish, tofu, or legumes, which supply essential amino acids for muscle repair and growth. And don't forget healthy fats from sources such as nuts, seeds, avocados, and olive oil, which support heart health and brain function.

Practical Tips for Meal Planning:

Meal planning is the key to success when it comes to creating balanced, delicious meals with ease. Start by setting aside time each week to plan your meals and create a shopping list, taking into account your dietary preferences, nutritional needs, and schedule. Consider batch cooking and meal prep on weekends to save time and streamline meal preparation during the week. Choose recipes that are simple, versatile, and adaptable to your taste preferences and ingredient availability. Experiment with different cooking techniques and flavour combinations to keep meals exciting and satisfying. And don't forget to stock your pantry with staple ingredients such as herbs, spices, whole grains, and canned or frozen fruits and vegetables, which can serve as the building blocks for a wide variety of meals.

Balanced Meal Ideas and Recipes:

Creating balanced meals doesn't have to be complicated or time-consuming. Here are some simple meal ideas and recipes to inspire your culinary creativity:

• Breakfast: Start your day with a balanced breakfast such as oatmeal topped with fresh berries, sliced almonds, and a drizzle of honey. Or try a smoothie made with spinach, banana, Greek yogurt, and a scoop of protein powder for a quick and nutritious option on busy mornings.

• Lunch: For a satisfying lunch, try a colourful salad filled with mixed greens, cherry tomatoes, cucumber, avocado, and grilled chicken or tofu. Dress it with a homemade vinaigrette made with olive oil, balsamic vinegar, Dijon mustard, and honey for a burst of flavor.

• Dinner: For a hearty and wholesome dinner, whip up a batch of vegetable stir-fry with tofu or shrimp, served over brown rice or quinoa. Or try a comforting bowl of vegetable soup made with hearty vegetables such as carrots, celery, and potatoes, simmered in a flavorful broth with herbs and spices.

Mindful Eating Habits:

In addition to creating balanced meals, it's important to practice mindful eating habits to fully enjoy and appreciate your food. Slow down and savour each bite, paying attention to the flavours, textures, and aromas of your meal. Chew your food thoroughly and take breaks between bites to give your body time to register feelings of fullness and satisfaction. Eat in a calm, relaxed environment free from distractions such as television or smartphones, allowing yourself to fully engage with the experience of eating. And listen to your body's hunger and fullness cues, stopping when you feel satisfied rather than overly full. By practicing mindful eating habits, you cultivate a deeper connection with your food and enhance the pleasure and satisfaction of eating.

Sample Meal Plans And Recipes To Inspire Your Culinary Journey.

Embarking on a journey towards healthier eating can be both exciting and daunting. However, with the right tools and inspiration, creating delicious and nutritious meals can become a rewarding and enjoyable part of your lifestyle. We will provide practical tips, sample meal plans, and flavorful recipes to ignite your culinary creativity and support your journey towards optimal health and well-being.

Practical Tips for Meal Planning:

Before diving into sample meal plans and recipes, let's review some practical tips for effective meal planning:

1. Set aside time for planning. Dedicate a specific time

each week to plan your meals and create a shopping list. Consider your schedule, dietary preferences, and nutritional needs when planning your meals.

2. Choose versatile ingredients: Opt for ingredients that can be used in multiple recipes to reduce waste and streamline meal preparation. Staples like whole grains, lean proteins, and fresh produce are versatile and can be incorporated into a variety of dishes.

3. Batch cooking and meal prepping: Spend some time on weekends batch cooking and meal prepping to save time during busy weekdays. Cook large batches of grains, proteins, and vegetables that can be used as the building blocks for multiple meals throughout the week.

4. Experiment with flavours and cuisines. Don't be afraid to get creative in the kitchen! Experiment with different herbs, spices, and cooking techniques to add depth and flavour to your meals. Explore cuisines from around the world to broaden your culinary horizons and discover new favorite dishes.

Sample Meal Plans:

Here are two sample meal plans to get you started on your culinary journey:

Sample Meal Plan 1:

Breakfast: avocado toast with whole grain bread, topped with sliced tomatoes, arugula, and a poached egg. Lunch: Quinoa salad with mixed greens, cherry tomatoes, cucumber, chickpeas, and feta cheese, dressed with a lemon vinaigrette. Dinner: Grilled salmon with roasted sweet potatoes and steamed broccoli. Snacks: Greek yoghurt with berries, sliced apples with almond butter.

Sample Meal Plan 2:

Breakfast: Overnight oats made with rolled oats, almond milk, chia seeds, and sliced bananas, topped with nuts and seeds. Lunch: whole grain wrap filled with hummus, sliced turkey or tofu, spinach, shredded carrots, and sliced avocado. Dinner: Vegetable stir-fry with tofu or shrimp, served over brown rice. Snacks: carrot sticks with hummus, mixed nuts, and apple slices with peanut butter.

Sample Recipes:

Here are two delicious recipes to try:

Recipe 1: Quinoa-Stuffed Bell Peppers

Ingredients:

• 4 large bell peppers, halved and seeded

• 1 cup of cooked quinoa

• 1 can black beans, drained and rinsed

• 1 cup of corn kernels (fresh or frozen)

• 1 cup diced tomatoes

• 1/2 cup chopped cilantro

• 1 teaspoon of cumin

• 1 teaspoon chilli powder

• Salt and pepper to taste

• Optional toppings: avocado, salsa, shredded cheese

Instructions:

1. Preheat the oven to 375°F (190°C). Place the bell pepper halves, cut-side up, in a baking dish.

2. In a large bowl, combine the cooked quinoa, black beans, corn, diced tomatoes, cilantro, cumin, chilli powder, salt, and pepper. Mix well to combine.

3. Spoon the quinoa mixture into each bell pepper half, pressing down gently to pack the filling.

4. Cover the baking dish with foil and bake for 25–30 minutes, or until the bell peppers are tender.

5. Remove from the oven and let cool slightly before serving. Top with avocado, salsa, and shredded cheese, if desired.

Recipe 2: Chickpea and Vegetable Curry

Ingredients:

• 1 tablespoon coconut oil or olive oil

• 1 onion, diced

• 2 cloves garlic, minced

• 1 tablespoon grated ginger

• 1 tablespoon curry powder

• 1 teaspoon ground cumin

• 1 teaspoon of ground turmeric

• 1 can chickpeas, drained and rinsed

• 2 cups diced vegetables (such as carrots, bell peppers,

zucchini, and cauliflower)

• 1 can of coconut milk

• Salt and pepper to taste

• Fresh cilantro for garnish

Instructions:

1. In a large skillet or pot, heat the coconut oil over medium heat. Add the diced onion, garlic, and ginger, and sauté until softened and fragrant, about 5 minutes.

2. Stir in the curry powder, cumin, and turmeric, and cook for an additional minute.

3. Add the chickpeas, diced vegetables, and coconut milk to the skillet, stirring to combine. Bring to a simmer, then reduce the heat to low and cover. Cook for 15-20 minutes, or until the vegetables are tender.

4. Season with salt and pepper to taste, and garnish with fresh cilantro before serving. Serve over cooked brown rice or quinoa, if desired.

CHAPTER TWO

Plant-Based Recipes

Veggie Stir-Fry with Tofu

Ingredients:

- 1 block (14 oz) extra-firm tofu, pressed and cubed
- 2 tablespoons of soy sauce
- 1 tablespoon sesame oil
- 1 tablespoon of cornflour
- 1 tablespoon of vegetable oil
- 2 cloves garlic, minced
- 1 tablespoon ginger, minced
- 1 onion, sliced
- 2 carrots, julienned
- 1 bell pepper, sliced
- 1 cup of broccoli florets
- 1 cup snap peas, trimmed
- 1 cup mushrooms, sliced
- 1/4 cup of vegetable broth
- 2 tablespoons of hoisin sauce

• Cooked brown rice or quinoa for serving

Servings: 4

Prep Time: 20 minutes

Cooking Time: 20 minutes

Instructions:

1. In a medium bowl, combine the cubed tofu, soy sauce, sesame oil, and cornstarch. Toss until the tofu is well coated, and set aside to marinate for 10–15 minutes.

2. Heat the vegetable oil in a large skillet or wok over medium-high heat. Add the marinated tofu cubes and cook until golden brown and crispy on all sides, about 5-7 minutes. Remove the tofu from the skillet and set it aside.

3. In the same skillet, add the minced garlic and ginger. Stir-fry for 1-2 minutes until fragrant.

4. Add the sliced onion, julienned carrots, sliced bell pepper, broccoli florets, snap peas, and sliced mushrooms to the skillet. Stir-fry for 5–6 minutes until the vegetables are tender-crisp.

5. Pour in the vegetable broth and hoisin sauce, stirring to combine. Cook for an additional 2–3 minutes until the sauce has thickened slightly.

6. Return the cooked tofu to the skillet and toss to coat with the sauce and vegetables.

7. Serve the veggie stir-fry with tofu hot over cooked brown rice or quinoa.

Nutritional information (per serving, without rice or quinoa):

• Calories: 240

- Protein: 14g

- Carbohydrates: 19g

- Fat: 12g

- Fibre: 6g

Sweet Potato and Black Bean Tacos

Ingredients:

- 2 medium sweet potatoes, peeled and diced

- 1 tablespoon of olive oil

- 1 teaspoon chilli powder

- 1/2 teaspoon ground cumin

- 1/2 teaspoon smoked paprika

- Salt and pepper to taste

- 1 can (15 oz) black beans, rinsed and drained

- 1 cup of corn kernels (fresh or frozen)

- 1/2 red onion, diced

- 2 cloves garlic, minced

- 1 jalapeño, seeded and minced (optional)

- 8 small corn or flour tortillas

- Optional toppings: avocado slices, diced tomatoes, shredded lettuce, cilantro, lime wedges, salsa, Greek yoghurt, or sour cream.

Servings: 4 (2 tacos per serving)

Prep Time: 15 minutes

Cooking Time: 20 minutes

Instructions:

1. Preheat the oven to 400°F (200°C). Place the diced sweet potatoes on a baking sheet and drizzle with olive oil. Sprinkle with chilli powder, cumin, smoked paprika, salt, and pepper. Toss to coat evenly.

2. Roast the sweet potatoes in the preheated oven for 20–25 minutes, or until tender and lightly browned, stirring halfway through.

3. While the sweet potatoes are roasting, heat a skillet over medium heat. Add the black beans, corn kernels, diced red onion, minced garlic, and minced jalapeño (if using) to the skillet. Cook for 5–6 minutes, stirring occasionally, until heated through and fragrant. Season with salt and pepper, to taste.

4. Warm the tortillas in a dry skillet or microwave until soft and pliable.

5. To assemble the tacos, divide the roasted sweet potatoes and black bean mixture evenly among the warmed tortillas. Top with optional toppings such as avocado slices, diced tomatoes, shredded lettuce, cilantro, lime wedges, salsa, Greek yoghurt, or sour cream.

6. Serve the sweet potato and black bean tacos immediately, and enjoy!

Nutritional information (per serving, without toppings):

• Calories: 360

• Protein: 12g

• Carbohydrates: 65g

• Fat: 7g

• Fibre: 10g

Eggplant Parmesan (using breadcrumbs sparingly)

Ingredients:

- 2 medium eggplants, sliced into 1/4-inch rounds

- Salt for sweating eggplant

- 1 cup whole wheat breadcrumbs

- 1/4 cup grated Parmesan cheese

- 2 eggs, beaten

- 2 cups of marinara sauce

- 1 cup shredded mozzarella cheese

- Fresh basil leaves for garnish

Servings: 6

Prep Time: 30 minutes

Cooking Time: 30 minutes

Instructions:

1. Preheat the oven to 375°F (190°C). Line a baking sheet with parchment paper.

2. Place the eggplant slices in a colander and sprinkle them generously with salt. Let them sit for 20–30 minutes to release excess moisture. Rinse the salt off and pat the eggplant slices dry with paper towels.

3. In a shallow dish, combine the whole wheat breadcrumbs and grated Parmesan cheese. Dip each eggplant slice into the beaten eggs, then coat them evenly with the breadcrumb mixture.

4. Place the breaded eggplant slices on the prepared baking sheet. Bake in the preheated oven for 15-20 minutes,

flipping halfway through, until golden brown and crispy.

5. Spread a thin layer of marinara sauce on the bottom of a 9x13-inch baking dish. Arrange half of the baked eggplant slices in a single layer over the sauce.

6. Top the eggplant slices with another layer of marinara sauce, followed by half of the shredded mozzarella cheese.

7. Repeat the layers with the remaining eggplant slices, marinara sauce, and mozzarella cheese.

8. Bake the eggplant Parmesan in the preheated oven for 20–25 minutes, or until the cheese is melted and bubbly.

9. Remove the eggplant Parmesan from the oven and let it cool for a few minutes before serving.

10. Garnish with fresh basil leaves before serving, if desired.

Nutritional information (per serving):

• Calories: 230

• Protein: 13g

• Carbohydrates: 25g

• Fat: 9g

• Fibre: 8g

Butternut Squash and Kale Salad with Maple-Dijon Dressing

Ingredients:

For the salad:

• 1 small butternut squash, peeled, seeded, and diced

• 1 tablespoon of olive oil

• Salt and pepper to taste

• 1 bunch of kale, stems removed, and leaves torn into bite-sized pieces

• 1/4 cup dried cranberries

• 1/4 cup toasted pecans, chopped

• 1/4 cup crumbled feta cheese (optional)

For the Maple-Dijon Dressing:

• 2 tablespoons of olive oil

• 1 tablespoon apple cider vinegar

• 1 tablespoon of pure maple syrup

• 1 teaspoon Dijon mustard

• Salt and pepper to taste

Servings: 4

Prep Time: 15 minutes

Cooking Time: 20 minutes

Instructions:

1. Preheat the oven to 400°F (200°C).

2. Place the diced butternut squash on a baking sheet. Drizzle with olive oil, and season with salt and pepper. Toss to coat evenly.

3. Roast the butternut squash in the preheated oven for 20–25 minutes, or until tender and caramelised, stirring halfway through.

4. While the butternut squash is roasting, prepare the kale by massaging it with a little olive oil for a few minutes to tenderize it.

5. In a small bowl, whisk together the ingredients for the Maple-Dijon Dressing: olive oil, apple cider vinegar, maple syrup, Dijon mustard, salt, and pepper. Set aside.

6. Once the butternut squash is done roasting, remove it from the oven and let it cool slightly.

7. In a large salad bowl, combine the massaged kale, roasted butternut squash, dried cranberries, toasted pecans, and crumbled feta cheese (if using).

8. Drizzle the maple-dijon dressing over the salad and toss until everything is evenly coated.

9. Serve the butternut squash and kale salad immediately, and enjoy!

Nutritional information (per serving, without feta cheese):

• Calories: 220

• Protein: 3g

• Carbohydrates: 28g

• Fat: 12g

• Fibre: 4g

Cauliflower Curry with Basmati Rice

Ingredients:

For the cauliflower curry:

• 1 head of cauliflower, cut into florets

• 1 tablespoon coconut oil or vegetable oil

• 1 onion, finely chopped

• 3 cloves garlic, minced

• 1 tablespoon grated ginger

- 2 tablespoons of curry powder
- 1 teaspoon of ground turmeric
- 1 teaspoon ground cumin
- 1 teaspoon ground coriander
- 1 can (14 oz) of coconut milk
- 1 can (14 oz) diced tomatoes
- Salt and pepper to taste
- Fresh cilantro for garnish

For the basmati rice:

- 1 cup basmati rice
- 2 cups of water
- 1/2 teaspoon salt

Servings: 4

Prep Time: 15 minutes

Cooking Time: 30 minutes

Instructions:

1. Rinse the basmati rice under cold water until the water runs clear. Drain well.

2. In a medium saucepan, combine the rinsed basmati rice, water, and salt. Bring to a boil over high heat, then reduce the heat to low, cover, and simmer for 15-20 minutes, or until the rice is tender and all the water has been absorbed. Remove from heat and let it sit, covered, for 5 minutes. Fluff the rice with a fork before serving.

3. While the rice is cooking, prepare the cauliflower curry. Heat the coconut oil or vegetable oil in a large skillet or pot

over medium heat.

4. Add the chopped onion to the skillet and cook for 3–4 minutes until softened.

5. Stir in the minced garlic and grated ginger, and cook for another 1-2 minutes until fragrant.

6. Add the curry powder, ground turmeric, ground cumin, and ground coriander to the skillet. Cook, stirring constantly, for 1 minute to toast the spices.

7. Add the cauliflower florets to the skillet and toss to coat them in the spice mixture.

8. Pour in the coconut milk and diced tomatoes (with juices). Season with salt and pepper, to taste.

9. Bring the mixture to a simmer, then reduce the heat to low and cover. Cook for 15-20 minutes, or until the cauliflower is tender and the sauce has thickened.

10. Serve the cauliflower curry hot over cooked basmati rice, garnished with fresh cilantro leaves.

Nutritional information (per serving):

• Calories: 330

• Protein: 7g

• Carbohydrates: 42g

• Fat: 16g

• Fibre: 6g

Zucchini Noodles with Pesto and Cherry Tomatoes

Ingredients:

For the Zucchini Noodles:

• 4 medium zucchinis

• 1 tablespoon of olive oil

• Salt and pepper to taste

For the pesto:

• 2 cups fresh basil leaves, packed

• 1/3 cup pine nuts or walnuts

• 2 cloves garlic, minced

• 1/2 cup grated Parmesan cheese (optional; omit for vegan version)

• 1/2 cup olive oil

• Salt and pepper to taste

Additional Toppings:

• 1 cup cherry tomatoes, halved

• Grated Parmesan cheese for garnish (optional)

• Fresh basil leaves for garnish

Servings: 4

Prep Time: 15 minutes

Cooking Time: 5 minutes

Instructions:

1. Using a spiralizer or vegetable peeler, create zucchini noodles (zoodles) from the zucchini. Set aside.

2. In a food processor or blender, combine the fresh basil leaves, pine nuts or walnuts, minced garlic, and grated Parmesan cheese (if using). Pulse until the ingredients are finely chopped.

3. With the food processor or blender running, slowly drizzle in the olive oil until the pesto reaches your desired

consistency. Season with salt and pepper to taste. Set aside.

4. Heat the olive oil in a large skillet over medium heat. Add the zucchini noodles to the skillet and sauté for 2-3 minutes, or until just tender. Season with salt and pepper, to taste.

5. Remove the skillet from the heat and toss the zucchini noodles with the prepared pesto until evenly coated.

6. Transfer the zucchini noodles to serving plates. Top with halved cherry tomatoes, and garnish with grated Parmesan cheese (if using) and fresh basil leaves.

7. Serve the zucchini noodles with pesto and cherry tomatoes immediately, and enjoy!

Nutritional Information (per serving, without Parmesan cheese):

• Calories: 230

• Protein: 4g

• Carbohydrates: 9g

• Fat: 21g

• Fibre: 3g

Quinoa-stuffed Portobello mushrooms

Ingredients:

For the Quinoa Stuffing:

• 1 cup quinoa, rinsed

• 2 cups of vegetable broth or water

• 1 tablespoon of olive oil

• 1 small onion, finely chopped

- 2 cloves garlic, minced

- 1 bell pepper, diced

- 1 zucchini, diced

- 1 teaspoon dried thyme

- 1 teaspoon dried oregano

- Salt and pepper to taste

- 1/4 cup grated Parmesan cheese (optional; omit for vegan version)

- 1/4 cup chopped fresh parsley

For the portobello mushrooms:

- 4 large Portobello mushrooms, stems removed

- 2 tablespoons of balsamic vinegar

- 2 tablespoons of olive oil

- Salt and pepper to taste

Servings: 4

Prep Time: 15 minutes

Cooking Time: 25 minutes

Instructions:

1. Preheat the oven to 375°F (190°C). Line a baking sheet with parchment paper.

2. In a medium saucepan, combine the quinoa and vegetable broth or water. Bring to a boil over high heat, then reduce the heat to low, cover, and simmer for 15 minutes, or until the quinoa is cooked and the liquid is absorbed. Remove from heat and let it sit, covered, for 5 minutes. Fluff the quinoa with a fork and set it aside.

3. While the quinoa is cooking, prepare the portobello mushrooms. In a small bowl, whisk together the balsamic vinegar and olive oil. Brush the mixture over both sides of the portobello mushrooms. Season with salt and pepper, to taste.

4. Place the mushrooms on the prepared baking sheet, gill side up. Bake in the preheated oven for 10–12 minutes, or until the mushrooms are tender.

5. While the mushrooms are baking, heat the olive oil in a large skillet over medium heat. Add the chopped onion and minced garlic to the skillet. Cook for 3–4 minutes until softened.

6. Stir in the diced bell pepper and zucchini. Cook for another 3–4 minutes until the vegetables are tender.

7. Add the cooked quinoa to the skillet with the sautéed vegetables. Season with dried thyme, dried oregano, salt, and pepper. Cook for 2–3 minutes to allow the flavours to meld together.

8. Remove the skillet from the heat and stir in the grated Parmesan cheese (if using) and chopped fresh parsley.

9. Once the Portobello mushrooms are done baking, remove them from the oven. Carefully spoon the quinoa stuffing into the centre of each mushroom.

10. Return the stuffed mushrooms to the oven and bake for an additional 5 minutes.

11. Serve the quinoa-stuffed Portobello mushrooms hot, and enjoy!

Nutritional Information (per serving, without Parmesan cheese):

- Calories: 310

- Protein: 9g

- Carbohydrates: 37g

- Fat: 15g

- Fibre: 6g

Vegan Pad Thai with Tofu

Ingredients:

For the Pad Thai Sauce:

- 1/4 cup soy sauce or tamari

- 2 tablespoons of rice vinegar

- 2 tablespoons of maple syrup or brown sugar

- 1 tablespoon of lime juice

- 1 tablespoon Sriracha sauce (adjust to taste)

- 1 clove garlic, minced

- 1 teaspoon grated ginger

- Salt to taste

For the Pad Thai:

- 8 oz. of rice noodles

- 2 tablespoons of vegetable oil

- 1 block (14 oz) firm tofu, pressed and cubed

- 1 red bell pepper, thinly sliced

- 1 carrot, julienned

- 2 cups of bean sprouts

- 4 green onions, sliced

- 1/4 cup chopped peanuts (optional)

- Fresh cilantro for garnish

- Lime wedges for serving

Servings: 4

Prep Time: 15 minutes

Cooking Time: 15 minutes

Instructions:

1. In a small bowl, whisk together all the ingredients for the Pad Thai sauce: soy sauce (or tamari), rice vinegar, maple syrup (or brown sugar), lime juice, Sriracha sauce, minced garlic, grated ginger, and salt. Set aside.

2. Cook the rice noodles according to the package instructions until al dente. Drain and rinse under cold water to prevent sticking. Set aside.

3. Heat 1 tablespoon of vegetable oil in a large skillet or wok over medium-high heat. Add the cubed tofu and cook until golden brown and crispy on all sides, about 5-7 minutes. Remove the tofu from the skillet and set it aside.

4. In the same skillet, add the remaining tablespoon of vegetable oil. Add the sliced red bell pepper and julienned carrot to the skillet. Stir-fry for 2-3 minutes until slightly softened.

5. Add the cooked rice noodles, bean sprouts, sliced green onions, and the prepared Pad Thai sauce to the skillet. Toss everything together until well combined and heated through.

6. Return the cooked tofu to the skillet and gently toss to incorporate it with the noodles and vegetables.

7. Remove the skillet from the heat and transfer the vegan pad Thai to serving plates. Garnish with chopped peanuts (if using), fresh cilantro, and lime wedges.

8. Serve the vegan pad Thai hot, and enjoy!

Nutritional information (per serving, without peanuts):

• Calories: 430

• Protein: 14g

• Carbohydrates: 61g

• Fat: 14g

• Fibre: 6g

Mediterranean Stuffed Peppers with Couscous
Ingredients:

For the stuffed peppers:

• 4 large bell peppers (any colour), halved, and seeds removed

• 1 cup couscous

• 2 cups of vegetable broth or water

• 2 tablespoons of olive oil

• 1 onion, diced

• 2 cloves garlic, minced

• 1 can (15 oz) chickpeas, rinsed and drained

• 1 cup cherry tomatoes, halved

• 1/2 cup Kalamata olives, pitted and chopped

• 1/4 cup fresh parsley, chopped

• 1/4 cup fresh mint, chopped

- 1 teaspoon dried oregano

- Salt and pepper to taste

- Optional: crumbled feta cheese for topping

Servings: 4

Prep Time: 15 minutes

Cooking Time: 25 minutes

Instructions:

1. Preheat the oven to 375°F (190°C). Lightly grease a baking dish large enough to hold the pepper halves.

2. In a medium saucepan, bring the vegetable broth or water to a boil. Stir in the couscous, cover, and remove from the heat. Let it sit for 5 minutes, then fluff it with a fork.

3. While the couscous is cooking, heat the olive oil in a large skillet over medium heat. Add the diced onion and minced garlic to the skillet. Cook for 3–4 minutes until softened.

4. Add the chickpeas, cherry tomatoes, chopped olives, chopped parsley, chopped mint, and dried oregano to the skillet. Cook for another 2–3 minutes until heated through. Season with salt and pepper, to taste.

5. Remove the skillet from the heat and stir in the cooked couscous until well combined.

6. Stuff each bell pepper half with the couscous mixture, pressing down gently to pack it in.

7. Place the stuffed peppers in the prepared baking dish. If desired, sprinkle crumbled feta cheese over the tops of the stuffed peppers.

8. Cover the baking dish with aluminium foil and bake in

the preheated oven for 20–25 minutes, or until the peppers are tender.

9. Remove the foil during the last 5 minutes of baking to allow the cheese to melt and bubble, if using.

10. Once the stuffed peppers are done baking, remove them from the oven and let them cool for a few minutes before serving.

11. Serve the Mediterranean-stuffed peppers with couscous hot and enjoy!

Nutritional information (per serving, without feta cheese):

• Calories: 380

• Protein: 12g

• Carbohydrates: 62g

• Fat: 9g

• Fibre: 12g

Black Bean and Corn Salad with Avocado
Ingredients:

• 1 can (15 oz) black beans, rinsed and drained

• 1 cup of corn kernels (fresh, canned, or frozen)

• 1 avocado, diced

• 1 red bell pepper, diced

• 1/2 red onion, finely chopped

• 1/4 cup chopped fresh cilantro

• 2 tablespoons of lime juice

• 2 tablespoons of olive oil

• 1 teaspoon ground cumin

• Salt and pepper to taste

Servings: 4

Prep Time: 10 minutes

Instructions:

1. In a large mixing bowl, combine the black beans, corn kernels, diced avocado, diced red bell pepper, finely chopped red onion, and chopped fresh cilantro.

2. In a small bowl, whisk together the lime juice, olive oil, ground cumin, salt, and pepper to make the dressing.

3. Pour the dressing over the black bean and corn mixture in the large mixing bowl. Toss gently until everything is evenly coated with the dressing.

4. Taste and adjust the seasoning, adding more salt, pepper, or lime juice if needed.

5. Serve the black bean and corn salad with avocado immediately, or refrigerate for at least 30 minutes to allow the flavours to meld together before serving.

Nutritional information (per serving):

• Calories: 250

• Protein: 9g

• Carbohydrates: 32g

• Fat: 12g

• Fibre: 10g

Tofu Scramble with Spinach and Tomatoes
Ingredients:

• 1 block (14 oz) firm tofu, drained and pressed

- 2 tablespoons of olive oil

- 1 small onion, diced

- 2 cloves garlic, minced

- 2 cups fresh spinach leaves, chopped

- 1 cup cherry tomatoes, halved

- 1/2 teaspoon ground turmeric

- 1/2 teaspoon ground cumin

- Salt and pepper to taste

- Optional: nutritional yeast for added flavour.

Servings: 2

Prep Time: 10 minutes

Cook Time: 15 minutes

Instructions:

1. Crumble the drained and pressed tofu into a bowl, using your hands or a fork, to resemble scrambled eggs.

2. In a large skillet, heat the olive oil over medium heat. Add the diced onion and minced garlic, and sauté until softened and fragrant, about 3–4 minutes.

3. Add the crumbled tofu to the skillet, spreading it out evenly. Allow it to cook undisturbed for a few minutes to brown slightly.

4. Stir in the chopped spinach and halved cherry tomatoes, and cook until the spinach is wilted and the tomatoes are softened, about 2–3 minutes.

5. Sprinkle the ground turmeric and ground cumin over the tofu mixture, and season with salt and pepper to taste.

Stir well to combine, ensuring that the spices are evenly distributed.

6. Continue to cook for another 2-3 minutes, stirring occasionally, until the tofu is heated through and any excess moisture has evaporated.

7. Taste the tofu scramble and adjust the seasoning if necessary. For added flavour, sprinkle with nutritional yeast, if desired.

8. Remove the skillet from the heat and serve the tofu scramble with spinach and tomatoes immediately.

Nutritional information (per serving):

• Calories: 250

• Protein: 18g

• Carbohydrates: 12g

• Fat: 16g

• Fibre: 5g

Lentil Shepherd's Pie
Ingredients:

For the lentil filling:

• 1 cup green or brown lentils, rinsed

• 2 cups of vegetable broth or water

• 1 tablespoon of olive oil

• 1 onion, diced

• 2 carrots, diced

• 2 celery stalks, diced

• 2 cloves garlic, minced

- 1 teaspoon dried thyme

- 1 teaspoon dried rosemary

- 1 cup of frozen peas

- Salt and pepper to taste

For the mashed potato topping:

- 4 large potatoes, peeled and cut into chunks

- 1/4 cup unsweetened plant-based milk (such as almond or soy milk)

- 2 tablespoons of vegan butter or olive oil

- Salt and pepper to taste

Servings: 4-6

Prep Time: 15 minutes

Cooking Time: 45 minutes

Instructions:

1. Preheat the oven to 375°F (190°C). Lightly grease a 9x13-inch baking dish.

2. In a medium saucepan, combine the lentils and vegetable broth or water. Bring to a boil over high heat, then reduce the heat to low, cover, and simmer for 20–25 minutes, or until the lentils are tender and the liquid is absorbed. Remove from heat and set aside.

3. While the lentils are cooking, place the peeled and chopped potatoes in a large pot and cover with water. Bring to a boil over high heat, then reduce the heat to medium-low and simmer for 15-20 minutes, or until the potatoes are fork-tender.

4. While the potatoes are cooking, heat the olive oil in

a large skillet over medium heat. Add the diced onion, carrots, and celery to the skillet. Cook for 5-7 minutes, stirring occasionally, until the vegetables are softened.

5. Add the minced garlic, dried thyme, and dried rosemary to the skillet. Cook for an additional 1-2 minutes until fragrant.

6. Stir in the cooked lentils and frozen peas, and cook for another 2-3 minutes until heated through. Season with salt and pepper, to taste.

7. Drain the cooked potatoes and transfer them to a large mixing bowl. Add the plant-based milk and vegan butter or olive oil. Mash the potatoes until smooth and creamy. Season with salt and pepper, to taste.

8. Transfer the lentil filling to the prepared baking dish, spreading it out evenly. Spoon the mashed potatoes over the lentil filling, smoothing it out with a spatula.

9. Bake the lentil shepherd's pie in the preheated oven for 25–30 minutes, or until the mashed potato topping is golden brown and the filling is bubbling around the edges.

10. Remove the baking dish from the oven and let it cool for a few minutes before serving.

11. Serve the Lentil Shepherd's Pie hot, and enjoy!

Nutritional Information (per serving, based on 4 servings):

• Calories: 400

• Protein: 15g

• Carbohydrates: 65g

• Fat: 8g

• Fibre: 12g

Greek Orzo Salad with Olives and Feta (use sparingly)

Ingredients:

For the orzo salad:

• 1 cup of orzo pasta

• 1/2 English cucumber, diced

• 1 cup cherry tomatoes, halved

• 1/2 cup Kalamata olives, pitted and halved

• 1/4 cup red onion, finely chopped

• 1/4 cup fresh parsley, chopped

• 2 tablespoons fresh dill, chopped

For the dressing:

• 3 tablespoons extra virgin olive oil

• 2 tablespoons of lemon juice

• 1 clove garlic, minced

• 1 teaspoon dried oregano

• Salt and pepper to taste

For Garnish:

• 1/4 cup crumbled feta cheese (use sparingly)

• Additional fresh parsley and dill for garnish

Servings: 4

Prep Time: 10 minutes

Cooking Time: 10 minutes

Instructions:

1. Cook the orzo pasta according to the package

instructions until al dente. Drain and rinse under cold water to stop the cooking process. Transfer the cooked orzo to a large mixing bowl.

2. Add the diced cucumber, halved cherry tomatoes, halved Kalamata olives, finely chopped red onion, chopped fresh parsley, and chopped fresh dill to the bowl with the cooked orzo.

3. In a small bowl, whisk together the extra virgin olive oil, lemon juice, minced garlic, dried oregano, salt, and pepper to make the dressing.

4. Pour the dressing over the orzo salad ingredients in the mixing bowl. Toss gently until everything is evenly coated with the dressing.

5. Taste the orzo salad and adjust the seasoning if necessary, adding more salt, pepper, or lemon juice if desired.

6. Transfer the Greek Orzo Salad to a serving platter or individual plates. Sprinkle the crumbled feta cheese sparingly over the top.

7. Garnish with additional fresh parsley and dill for a pop of colour and flavour.

8. Serve the Greek Orzo Salad with Olives and Feta immediately, and enjoy!

Nutritional Information (per serving, with sparingly used feta cheese):

• Calories: 280

• Protein: 7g

• Carbohydrates: 32g

- Fat: 14g

- Fibre: 3g

Moroccan Chickpea Stew

Ingredients:

- 2 tablespoons of olive oil

- 1 onion, diced

- 2 cloves garlic, minced

- 1 teaspoon ground cumin

- 1 teaspoon ground coriander

- 1 teaspoon ground paprika

- 1/2 teaspoon ground turmeric

- 1/4 teaspoon ground cinnamon

- 1/4 teaspoon cayenne pepper (adjust to taste)

- 1 can (14 oz) diced tomatoes

- 2 cups of vegetable broth

- 2 cups cooked chickpeas (or 1 can, drained and rinsed)

- 2 cups chopped carrots

- 1 cup chopped bell peppers (any colour)

- 1 cup of chopped zucchini

- 1/4 cup chopped dried apricots

- Salt and pepper to taste

- Fresh cilantro or parsley for garnish

Servings: 4

Prep Time: 10 minutes

Cooking Time: 30 minutes

Instructions:

1. Heat the olive oil in a large pot or Dutch oven over medium heat. Add the diced onion and minced garlic, and sauté until softened and fragrant, about 3–4 minutes.

2. Stir in the ground cumin, ground coriander, ground paprika, ground turmeric, ground cinnamon, and cayenne pepper. Cook for another 1-2 minutes until the spices are toasted and aromatic.

3. Add the diced tomatoes (with their juices) and vegetable broth to the pot. Stir to combine, scraping up any browned bits from the bottom of the pot.

4. Add the cooked chickpeas, chopped carrots, chopped bell peppers, chopped zucchini, and chopped dried apricots to the pot. Stir well to combine.

5. Bring the stew to a simmer, then reduce the heat to low and cover. Let the stew simmer for 20–25 minutes, or until the vegetables are tender and the flavours have melded together.

6. Taste the stew and season with salt and pepper to taste, adjusting the seasoning as needed.

7. Ladle the Moroccan chickpea stew into serving bowls. Garnish with fresh cilantro or parsley before serving.

8. Serve the Moroccan chickpea stew hot, and enjoy!

Nutritional information (per serving):

• Calories: 280

• Protein: 9g

• Carbohydrates: 42g

• Fat: 9g

• Fibre: 11g

Roasted Vegetable and Hummus Wrap

Ingredients:

For the roasted vegetables:

• 1 small eggplant, diced

• 1 zucchini, diced

• 1 red bell pepper, sliced

• 1 yellow bell pepper, sliced

• 1 tablespoon of olive oil

• Salt and pepper to taste

• Optional: other favorite vegetables like cherry tomatoes or red onion slices

For the wrap:

• 4 whole wheat or spinach tortillas

• 1 cup hummus (store-bought or homemade)

• A handful of baby spinach leaves

• Optional: crumbled feta cheese (use sparingly)

• Optional: fresh herbs like parsley or cilantro for garnish.

Servings: 4

Prep Time: 15 minutes

Cooking Time: 20 minutes

Instructions:

1. Preheat the oven to 400°F (200°C). Line a baking sheet with parchment paper or lightly grease it.

2. In a large mixing bowl, toss together the diced eggplant, diced zucchini, sliced red bell pepper, sliced yellow bell pepper, and any other desired vegetables with olive oil, salt, and pepper until evenly coated.

3. Spread the seasoned vegetables in a single layer on the prepared baking sheet. Roast in the preheated oven for 15-20 minutes, or until the vegetables are tender and slightly caramelised, stirring halfway through cooking.

4. While the vegetables are roasting, warm the tortillas in a dry skillet over medium heat for about 30 seconds on each side, or until they are soft and pliable.

5. To assemble the wraps, spread a generous layer of hummus onto each tortilla, leaving a border around the edges.

6. Top the hummus with a handful of baby spinach leaves, followed by a portion of the roasted vegetables.

7. If desired, sprinkle a small amount of crumbled feta cheese sparingly over the vegetables for added flavour.

8. Garnish with fresh herbs like parsley or cilantro, if desired.

9. Roll up the wraps tightly, tucking in the sides as you go, to enclose the filling.

10. Slice the wraps in half diagonally, if desired, and serve immediately.

Nutritional information (per serving, without feta cheese):

• Calories: 320

• Protein: 10g

• Carbohydrates: 42g

- Fat: 12g
- Fibre: 10g

CHAPTER THREE

Low-Fat Recipes

Turkey Meatball Subs with Marinara Sauce (use lean turkey meat)

Ingredients:

For the turkey meatballs:

- 1 lb. lean ground turkey

- 1/4 cup of breadcrumbs

- 1/4 cup grated Parmesan cheese

- 1 egg

- 2 cloves garlic, minced

- 1 tablespoon chopped fresh parsley

- 1/2 teaspoon dried oregano

- 1/2 teaspoon dried basil

- Salt and pepper to taste

For the Marinara Sauce:

- 1 can (14 oz) crushed tomatoes

- 1/2 onion, finely chopped

- 2 cloves garlic, minced

- 1 tablespoon of olive oil

- 1 teaspoon dried basil

- 1 teaspoon dried oregano

- Salt and pepper to taste

For Assembling:

- 4 whole wheat sub rolls

- Shredded mozzarella cheese (optional)

- Chopped fresh parsley for garnish (optional)

Servings: 4

Prep Time: 15 minutes

Cook Time: 25 minutes

Instructions:

1. Preheat the oven to 400°F (200°C). Line a baking sheet with parchment paper, or lightly grease it with olive oil.

2. In a large mixing bowl, combine the lean ground turkey, breadcrumbs, grated Parmesan cheese, egg, minced garlic, chopped fresh parsley, dried oregano, dried basil, salt, and pepper. Mix until well combined.

3. Shape the turkey mixture into meatballs, about 1 inch in diameter, and place them on the prepared baking sheet.

4. Bake the turkey meatballs in the preheated oven for 15-20 minutes, or until they are cooked through and lightly browned on the outside.

5. While the meatballs are baking, prepare the marinara sauce. Heat the olive oil in a saucepan over medium heat. Add the finely chopped onion and minced garlic, and sauté for 2-3 minutes until softened and fragrant.

6. Add the crushed tomatoes, dried basil, dried oregano,

salt, and pepper to the saucepan. Stir well to combine.

7. Bring the marinara sauce to a simmer, then reduce the heat to low. Let it simmer for 10–15 minutes, stirring occasionally, to allow the flavours to meld together.

8. Once the turkey meatballs are done baking and the marinara sauce is ready, assemble the subs. Place the cooked meatballs in the whole wheat sub rolls and spoon marinara sauce over the top.

9. If desired, sprinkle shredded mozzarella cheese over the meatballs and marinara sauce.

10. Place the assembled subs back in the oven for a few minutes to melt the cheese and warm the rolls.

11. Garnish with chopped fresh parsley before serving, if desired.

Nutritional information (per serving, excluding optional cheese and garnish):

• Calories: 350

• Protein: 25g

• Carbohydrates: 35g

• Fat: 12g

• Fibre: 5g

Baked Sweet Potato Fries

Ingredients:

• 2 large sweet potatoes, peeled

• 2 tablespoons of olive oil

• 1 teaspoon paprika

• 1/2 teaspoon garlic powder

• 1/2 teaspoon onion powder

• 1/2 teaspoon dried thyme

• Salt and pepper to taste

• Optional: chopped fresh parsley for garnish.

Servings: 4

Prep Time: 10 minutes

Cook Time: 20 minutes

Instructions:

1. Preheat the oven to 425°F (220°C). Line a baking sheet with parchment paper or aluminium foil for easy cleanup.

2. Cut the peeled sweet potatoes into evenly-sized fries or wedges. Try to make them as uniform in size as possible for even baking.

3. In a large mixing bowl, toss the sweet potato fries with olive oil, paprika, garlic powder, onion powder, dried thyme, salt, and pepper until evenly coated.

4. Spread the seasoned sweet potato fries in a single layer on the prepared baking sheet, making sure they are not overcrowded. Use two baking sheets if necessary to avoid overcrowding.

5. Bake the sweet potato fries in the preheated oven for 15-20 minutes, flipping halfway through cooking, until they are golden brown and crispy on the outside and tender on the inside.

6. Once the sweet potato fries are done baking, remove them from the oven and let them cool for a few minutes before serving.

7. Garnish with chopped fresh parsley for added colour and

flavour, if desired.

8. Serve the baked sweet potato fries hot as a delicious and nutritious side dish or snack.

Nutritional information (per serving):

• Calories: 150

• Protein: 2g

• Carbohydrates: 20g

• Fat: 7g

• Fibre: 3g

Grilled Chicken Caesar Salad (use a light dressing)
Ingredients:

For the grilled chicken:

• 2 boneless, skinless chicken breasts

• 1 tablespoon of olive oil

• 1 teaspoon garlic powder

• 1 teaspoon dried oregano

• Salt and pepper to taste

For the Caesar Salad:

• 1 head of romaine lettuce, washed and chopped

• 1/4 cup grated Parmesan cheese

• 1/2 cup croutons (optional)

• Lemon wedges for garnish (optional)

For the Light Caesar Dressing:

• 1/4 cup non-fat Greek yoghurt

- 1 tablespoon Dijon mustard

- 1 tablespoon of lemon juice

- 1 tablespoon grated Parmesan cheese

- 1 clove garlic, minced

- 1 teaspoon Worcestershire sauce

- Salt and pepper to taste

Servings: 2

Prep Time: 15 minutes

Cook Time: 15 minutes

Instructions:

1. Preheat the grill to medium-high heat.

2. In a small bowl, mix together the olive oil, garlic powder, dried oregano, salt, and pepper to make a marinade for the chicken.

3. Brush the marinade over the chicken breasts, ensuring they are evenly coated on both sides.

4. Grill the chicken breasts on the preheated grill for 6–8 minutes per side, or until they are cooked through and have grill marks. The internal temperature should reach 165°F (74°C). Remove the chicken from the grill and let it rest for a few minutes before slicing.

5. While the chicken is grilling, prepare the Caesar salad dressing. In a small bowl, whisk together the non-fat Greek yoghurt, Dijon mustard, lemon juice, grated Parmesan cheese, minced garlic, Worcestershire sauce, salt, and pepper until smooth and well combined.

6. In a large salad bowl, combine the chopped romaine

lettuce, grated Parmesan cheese, and croutons (if using).

7. Once the chicken has rested, slice it thinly against the grain.

8. Add the sliced, grilled chicken to the salad bowl.

9. Drizzle the light Caesar dressing over the salad and toss until everything is evenly coated.

10. Divide the grilled chicken Caesar salad between serving plates.

11. Garnish with lemon wedges for extra flavour, if desired.

Nutritional information (per serving):

• Calories: 300

• Protein: 35g

• Carbohydrates: 15g

• Fat: 12g

• Fibre: 5g

Quinoa-Stuffed Bell Peppers with Ground Turkey

Ingredients:

For the Stuffed Bell Peppers:

• 4 large bell peppers (any color), tops removed and seeds removed

• 1 cup quinoa, rinsed

• 1 lb. lean ground turkey

• 1 tablespoon of olive oil

• 1 onion, finely chopped

• 2 cloves garlic, minced

- 1 can (15 oz) diced tomatoes, drained

- 1 teaspoon ground cumin

- 1 teaspoon paprika

- Salt and pepper to taste

- 1/2 cup shredded mozzarella cheese (optional)

For Garnish:

- Chopped fresh parsley or cilantro

- Lemon wedges (optional)

Servings: 4

Prep Time: 15 minutes

Cook Time: 35 minutes

Instructions:

1. Preheat the oven to 375°F (190°C). Lightly grease a baking dish large enough to hold the stuffed bell peppers.

2. In a medium saucepan, bring 2 cups of water to a boil. Add the rinsed quinoa, reduce the heat to low, cover, and simmer for 15-20 minutes, or until the quinoa is cooked and the water is absorbed. Remove from heat and set aside.

3. In a large skillet, heat the olive oil over medium heat. Add the finely chopped onion and minced garlic, and cook for 3–4 minutes until softened and fragrant.

4. Add the lean, ground turkey to the skillet, breaking it apart with a spoon. Cook for 5–6 minutes, stirring occasionally, until the turkey is browned and cooked through.

5. Stir in the drained diced tomatoes, ground cumin, paprika, cooked quinoa, salt, and pepper. Cook for another

2–3 minutes to allow the flavours to meld together. Remove from heat.

6. Stuff each hollowed-out bell pepper with the turkey and quinoa mixture, pressing down gently to fill it completely.

7. Place the stuffed bell peppers in the prepared baking dish. If using shredded mozzarella cheese, sprinkle it over the tops of the stuffed peppers.

8. Cover the baking dish with aluminium foil and bake in the preheated oven for 25–30 minutes, or until the peppers are tender.

9. Remove the foil and continue baking for an additional 5–10 minutes, or until the cheese is melted and bubbly (if using).

10. Once the stuffed bell peppers are done baking, remove them from the oven and let them cool for a few minutes before serving.

11. Garnish with chopped fresh parsley or cilantro, and serve hot with lemon wedges on the side, if desired.

Nutritional information (per serving, without optional cheese):

· Calories: 350

· Protein: 30g

· Carbohydrates: 35g

· Fat: 10g

· Fibre: 7g

Baked eggplant parmesan (use minimal cheese)
Ingredients:

· 1 large eggplant, sliced into 1/2-inch rounds

- 1 cup whole wheat breadcrumbs
- 2 eggs, beaten
- 1/4 cup grated Parmesan cheese
- 1 teaspoon dried oregano
- 1 teaspoon dried basil
- 1/2 teaspoon garlic powder
- Salt and pepper to taste
- Olive oil cooking spray
- 1 cup of marinara sauce
- 1/2 cup shredded, part-skim mozzarella cheese
- Fresh basil leaves for garnish (optional)

Servings: 4

Prep Time: 20 minutes

Cook Time: 25 minutes

Instructions:

1. Preheat the oven to 400°F (200°C). Line a baking sheet with parchment paper, or lightly grease it with olive oil.

2. In a shallow dish, combine the whole wheat breadcrumbs, grated Parmesan cheese, dried oregano, dried basil, garlic powder, salt, and pepper.

3. Dip each eggplant slice into the beaten eggs, then coat both sides with the breadcrumb mixture. Press gently to adhere the breadcrumbs to the eggplant.

4. Place the breaded eggplant slices on the prepared baking sheet in a single layer.

5. Lightly spray the tops of the breaded eggplant slices with

olive oil cooking spray.

6. Bake in the preheated oven for 15–20 minutes, flipping halfway through cooking, until the eggplant is golden brown and tender.

7. Remove the baked eggplant slices from the oven and reduce the oven temperature to 350°F (175°C).

8. In a baking dish, spread a thin layer of marinara sauce on the bottom.

9. Arrange the baked eggplant slices in the baking dish in a single layer, slightly overlapping if necessary.

10. Top each eggplant slice with a spoonful of marinara sauce and a sprinkle of shredded, part-skim mozzarella cheese.

11. Bake in the oven at 350°F (175°C) for an additional 10–15 minutes, or until the cheese is melted and bubbly.

12. Once done, remove it from the oven and let it cool for a few minutes before serving.

13. Garnish with fresh basil leaves if desired, and serve hot.

Nutritional information (per serving):

• Calories: 200

• Protein: 10g

• Carbohydrates: 25g

• Fat: 6g

• Fibre: 7g

Turkey Taco Lettuce Wraps
Ingredients:

For the turkey taco filling:

- 1 lb. lean ground turkey
- 1 tablespoon of olive oil
- 1 onion, diced
- 2 cloves garlic, minced
- 1 bell pepper, diced (any colour)
- 1 can (15 oz) black beans, drained and rinsed
- 1 cup of corn kernels (fresh, canned, or frozen)
- 1 tablespoon chilli powder
- 1 teaspoon ground cumin
- 1/2 teaspoon paprika
- Salt and pepper to taste
- 1/4 cup chopped fresh cilantro
- Juice of 1 lime

For Assembling:

- Large lettuce leaves (such as romaine or butter lettuce)
- Optional toppings: diced tomatoes, diced avocado, shredded cheese, Greek yoghurt or sour cream, salsa, hot sauce

Servings: 4

Prep Time: 10 minutes

Cook Time: 15 minutes

Instructions:

1. Heat the olive oil in a large skillet over medium heat. Add the diced onion and minced garlic, and sauté for 2-3 minutes until softened and fragrant.

2. Add the lean, ground turkey to the skillet, breaking it apart with a spoon. Cook for 5–6 minutes, stirring occasionally, until the turkey is browned and cooked through.

3. Add the diced bell pepper, black beans, and corn kernels to the skillet with the cooked turkey. Stir in the chilli powder, ground cumin, paprika, salt, and pepper.

4. Cook for another 4-5 minutes, stirring occasionally, until the bell pepper is tender and the flavors are well combined.

5. Remove the skillet from the heat and stir in the chopped fresh cilantro and lime juice. Taste and adjust the seasoning if necessary.

6. To assemble the lettuce wraps, spoon a generous amount of the turkey taco filling onto each lettuce leaf.

7. Top the turkey taco filling with your favourite toppings, such as diced tomatoes, diced avocado, shredded cheese, Greek yoghurt or sour cream, salsa, and hot sauce.

8. Roll up the lettuce leaves to enclose the filling, securing them with toothpicks if necessary.

9. Serve the turkey taco lettuce wraps immediately, with extra toppings on the side if desired.

Nutritional information (per serving, excluding optional toppings):

• Calories: 250

• Protein: 25g

• Carbohydrates: 20g

• Fat: 8g

• Fibre: 6g

Grilled Shrimp and Vegetable Skewers

Ingredients:

For the Marinade:

• 1/4 cup olive oil

• 2 cloves garlic, minced

• 2 tablespoons of lemon juice

• 1 teaspoon lemon zest

• 1 tablespoon chopped fresh parsley

• 1 teaspoon dried oregano

• 1/2 teaspoon paprika

• Salt and pepper to taste

For the Skewers:

• 1 lb. large shrimp, peeled and deveined

• 1 red bell pepper, cut into chunks

• 1 yellow bell pepper, cut into chunks

• 1 red onion, cut into chunks

• 1 zucchini, sliced into rounds

• 8-10 cherry tomatoes

• Wooden skewers, soaked in water for at least 30 minutes

Servings: 4

Prep Time: 20 minutes

Marinating Time: 30 minutes

Cook Time: 8–10 minutes

Instructions:

1. In a small bowl, whisk together the olive oil, minced garlic, lemon juice, lemon zest, chopped fresh parsley, dried oregano, paprika, salt, and pepper to make the marinade.

2. Place the peeled and deveined shrimp in a large resealable plastic bag or shallow dish. Pour the marinade over the shrimp, making sure they are evenly coated. Seal the bag or cover the dish, and refrigerate for at least 30 minutes to marinate.

3. Preheat the grill to medium-high heat.

4. While the shrimp is marinating, prepare the vegetables. Cut the red and yellow bell peppers, red onion, zucchini, and cherry tomatoes into chunks or slices, depending on your preference.

5. Remove the shrimp from the marinade, reserving any excess marinade.

6. Thread the marinated shrimp and prepared vegetables onto the soaked wooden skewers, alternating between shrimp and vegetables.

7. Brush the skewers with the reserved marinade for extra flavour.

8. Place the skewers on the preheated grill and cook for 3–4 minutes per side, or until the shrimp are pink and opaque and the vegetables are tender and lightly charred.

9. Once done, remove the skewers from the grill and serve immediately.

10. Optionally, garnish the grilled shrimp and vegetable skewers with additional chopped fresh parsley or a squeeze of lemon juice before serving.

Nutritional information (per serving):

- Calories: 250

- Protein: 25g

- Carbohydrates: 12g

- Fat: 12g

- Fibre: 3g

Oven-Baked Chicken Fajitas

Ingredients:

For the Chicken and Marinade:

- 1 lb. boneless, skinless chicken breasts, thinly sliced

- 2 tablespoons of olive oil

- 2 tablespoons of lime juice

- 1 teaspoon chilli powder

- 1 teaspoon ground cumin

- 1/2 teaspoon smoked paprika

- 1/2 teaspoon garlic powder

- Salt and pepper to taste

For the Fajita Vegetables:

- 1 red bell pepper, thinly sliced

- 1 green bell pepper, thinly sliced

- 1 yellow onion, thinly sliced

For Serving:

- 8 small whole wheat tortillas

- Optional toppings: diced tomatoes, shredded lettuce, diced avocado, shredded cheese, Greek yoghurt or sour cream, salsa, hot sauce

Servings: 4

Prep Time: 15 minutes

Marinating Time: 30 minutes

Cook Time: 20 minutes

Instructions:

1. In a large mixing bowl, combine the olive oil, lime juice, chilli powder, ground cumin, smoked paprika, garlic powder, salt, and pepper to make the marinade.

2. Add the thinly sliced chicken breasts to the marinade and toss until evenly coated. Cover the bowl and refrigerate for at least 30 minutes to marinate.

3. Preheat the oven to 400°F (200°C). Line a baking sheet with parchment paper or aluminium foil for easy cleanup.

4. Spread the sliced bell peppers and onion on the prepared baking sheet.

5. Remove the chicken from the marinade and add it to the baking sheet with the vegetables, spreading everything out in an even layer.

6. Bake in the preheated oven for 15-20 minutes, or until the chicken is cooked through and the vegetables are tender and slightly caramelized.

7. While the chicken and vegetables are baking, warm the whole wheat tortillas according to package instructions.

8. Once done, remove the baking sheet from the oven and serve the oven-baked chicken fajitas immediately with warmed tortillas and your choice of toppings.

9. Let everyone assemble their own fajitas by filling the tortillas with the baked chicken and vegetables and adding

toppings as desired.

Nutritional information (per serving, excluding toppings):

• Calories: 300

• Protein: 25g

• Carbohydrates: 30g

• Fat: 10g

• Fibre: 5g

Lemon-Garlic Shrimp with Brown Rice
Ingredients:

For the Lemon-Garlic Shrimp:

• 1 lb. large shrimp, peeled and deveined

• 2 tablespoons of olive oil

• 4 cloves garlic, minced

• Zest of 1 lemon

• Juice of 1 lemon

• 1 teaspoon dried oregano

• Salt and pepper to taste

• Chopped fresh parsley for garnish

For the brown rice:

• 1 cup of brown rice

• 2 cups water or vegetable broth

• Salt to taste

Servings: 4

Prep Time: 10 minutes

Cook Time: 20 minutes

Instructions:

1. Rinse the brown rice under cold water until the water runs clear. Drain well.

2. In a medium saucepan, combine the rinsed brown rice and water or vegetable broth. Add salt to taste. Bring to a boil over high heat.

3. Reduce the heat to low, cover, and simmer for 18–20 minutes, or until the rice is tender and all the liquid is absorbed. Remove from heat and let it sit, covered, for 5 minutes. Fluff the rice with a fork before serving.

4. While the rice is cooking, prepare the lemon-garlic shrimp. In a large skillet, heat the olive oil over medium heat.

5. Add the minced garlic to the skillet and sauté for 1-2 minutes until fragrant.

6. Add the peeled and deveined shrimp to the skillet in a single layer. Cook for 2-3 minutes per side, or until the shrimp turns pink and opaque.

7. Add the lemon zest, lemon juice, dried oregano, salt, and pepper to the skillet with the cooked shrimp. Stir well to coat the shrimp evenly in the lemon-garlic sauce.

8. Cook for another 1-2 minutes, allowing the flavours to meld together.

9. Once done, remove the skillet from the heat.

10. Serve the lemon-garlic shrimp hot over cooked brown rice.

11. Garnish with chopped fresh parsley before serving.

Nutritional information (per serving):

• Calories: 300

• Protein: 25g

• Carbohydrates: 30g

• Fat: 10g

• Fibre: 3g

Turkey and Vegetable Kabobs

Ingredients:

For the Turkey Marinade:

• 1 lb. lean turkey breast, cut into 1-inch cubes

• 2 tablespoons of olive oil

• 2 tablespoons soy sauce (or tamari for a gluten-free option)

• 2 cloves garlic, minced

• 1 teaspoon dried oregano

• 1 teaspoon paprika

• 1/2 teaspoon ground cumin

• Salt and pepper to taste

For the vegetable kabobs:

• 2 bell peppers (any colour), cut into chunks

• 1 red onion, cut into chunks

• 1 zucchini, sliced into rounds

• 1 pint of cherry tomatoes

• Wooden skewers, soaked in water for at least 30 minutes

Servings: 4

Prep Time: 20 minutes

Marinating Time: 30 minutes

Cook Time: 10–12 minutes

Instructions:

1. In a large mixing bowl, combine the olive oil, soy sauce, minced garlic, dried oregano, paprika, ground cumin, salt, and pepper to make the marinade for the turkey.

2. Add the cubed turkey breast to the marinade and toss until evenly coated. Cover the bowl and refrigerate for at least 30 minutes to marinate.

3. While the turkey is marinating, prepare the vegetables. Cut the bell peppers, red onion, and zucchini into chunks or slices, depending on your preference.

4. Preheat the grill to medium-high heat.

5. Remove the turkey from the marinade and discard any excess marinade. Thread the marinated turkey cubes and prepared vegetables onto the soaked wooden skewers, alternating between turkey and vegetables.

6. Place the assembled turkey and vegetable kabobs on the preheated grill.

7. Grill the kabobs for 5–6 minutes per side, or until the turkey is cooked through and the vegetables are tender and slightly charred.

8. Once done, remove the turkey and vegetable kabobs from the grill and serve immediately.

9. Optionally, garnish with chopped fresh parsley or a squeeze of lemon juice before serving.

Note: You can also cook the kabobs in the oven under the broiler for 10–12 minutes, flipping halfway through cooking, if you prefer.

Nutritional information (per serving):

• Calories: 250

• Protein: 30g

• Carbohydrates: 15g

• Fat: 8g

• Fibre: 4g

Baked Chicken Tenders with Honey Mustard Sauce (use sparingly)

Ingredients:

For the baked chicken tenders:

• 1 lb. chicken breast tenders (or chicken breast cut into strips)

• 1 cup whole wheat breadcrumbs

• 2 tablespoons grated Parmesan cheese

• 1 teaspoon garlic powder

• 1 teaspoon paprika

• Salt and pepper to taste

• 2 eggs, beaten

For the Honey Mustard Sauce:

• 2 tablespoons Dijon mustard

• 1 tablespoon of honey

• 1 tablespoon Greek yoghurt (or mayonnaise)

• 1 teaspoon of lemon juice

• Salt and pepper to taste

Servings: 4

Prep Time: 15 minutes

Cook Time: 15 minutes

Instructions:

1. Preheat the oven to 400°F (200°C). Line a baking sheet with parchment paper, or lightly grease it with olive oil.

2. In a shallow dish, combine the whole wheat breadcrumbs, grated Parmesan cheese, garlic powder, paprika, salt, and pepper.

3. Dip each chicken tender into the beaten eggs, then coat both sides with the breadcrumb mixture. Press gently to adhere the breadcrumbs to the chicken.

4. Place the breaded chicken tenders on the prepared baking sheet in a single layer.

5. Bake in the preheated oven for 12–15 minutes, flipping halfway through cooking, until the chicken is golden brown and cooked through.

6. While the chicken tenders are baking, prepare the honey mustard sauce. In a small bowl, whisk together the Dijon mustard, honey, Greek yoghurt (or mayonnaise), lemon juice, salt, and pepper until smooth and well combined.

7. Once the chicken tenders are done baking, remove them from the oven and let them cool for a few minutes.

8. Serve the baked chicken tenders hot with the honey mustard sauce on the side for dipping.

Nutritional information (per serving, including sauce):

- Calories: 250

- Protein: 30g

- Carbohydrates: 15g

- Fat: 8g

- Fibre: 2g

Turkey and Black Bean Enchiladas (use low-fat cheese)
Ingredients:

For the enchilada filling:

- 1 lb. lean ground turkey

- 1 tablespoon of olive oil

- 1 onion, diced

- 2 cloves garlic, minced

- 1 bell pepper, diced

- 1 can (15 oz) black beans, drained and rinsed

- 1 cup of corn kernels (fresh, canned, or frozen)

- 1 teaspoon ground cumin

- 1 teaspoon chilli powder

- Salt and pepper to taste

- 1/4 cup chopped fresh cilantro

- 8 whole wheat tortillas

For the Enchilada Sauce:

- 2 cups of tomato sauce

- 1 cup of low-sodium chicken broth

- 2 cloves garlic, minced

- 1 teaspoon ground cumin

- 1 teaspoon chilli powder

- Salt and pepper to taste

For Topping:

- 1 cup shredded low-fat cheese (such as cheddar or Mexican blend)

- Chopped fresh cilantro

- Diced avocado

- Greek yoghurt or sour cream (optional)

Servings: 4

Prep Time: 20 minutes

Cook Time: 25 minutes

Instructions:

1. Preheat the oven to 375°F (190°C). Lightly grease a 9x13-inch baking dish with olive oil or non-stick cooking spray.

2. In a large skillet, heat the olive oil over medium heat. Add the diced onion and minced garlic, and sauté for 2-3 minutes until softened and fragrant.

3. Add the lean, ground turkey to the skillet, breaking it apart with a spoon. Cook for 5–6 minutes, stirring occasionally, until the turkey is browned and cooked through.

4. Stir in the diced bell pepper, drained black beans, corn kernels, ground cumin, chilli powder, salt, and pepper. Cook for another 4-5 minutes, until the bell pepper is tender and the flavours are well combined. Remove from heat and stir in the chopped fresh cilantro.

5. To make the enchilada sauce, in a separate saucepan, combine the tomato sauce, low-sodium chicken broth, minced garlic, ground cumin, chilli powder, salt, and pepper. Bring to a simmer over medium heat and cook for 5-7 minutes, stirring occasionally, until the sauce has thickened slightly. Remove from heat.

6. To assemble the enchiladas, spoon a generous amount of the turkey and black bean filling onto each whole wheat tortilla. Roll up the tortillas and place them seam-side down in the prepared baking dish.

7. Pour the enchilada sauce evenly over the rolled tortillas in the baking dish.

8. Sprinkle the shredded low-fat cheese over the top of the enchiladas.

9. Cover the baking dish with aluminium foil and bake in the preheated oven for 20 minutes.

10. Remove the foil and bake for an additional 5 minutes, or until the cheese is melted and bubbly.

11. Once done, remove the enchiladas from the oven and let them cool for a few minutes before serving.

12. Garnish with chopped fresh cilantro and diced avocado, and serve hot with Greek yoghurt or sour cream on the side, if desired.

Nutritional information (per serving):

• Calories: 400

• Protein: 30g

• Carbohydrates: 45g

• Fat: 12g

• Fibre: 10g

Grilled Lemon-Herb Chicken Breast

Ingredients:

For the Lemon-Herb Marinade:

• 4 boneless, skinless chicken breasts

• 1/4 cup olive oil

• Zest of 1 lemon

• Juice of 1 lemon

• 2 cloves garlic, minced

• 2 tablespoons chopped fresh parsley

• 1 tablespoon chopped fresh thyme (or 1 teaspoon dried thyme)

• 1 tablespoon chopped fresh rosemary (or 1 teaspoon dried rosemary)

• Salt and pepper to taste

Servings: 4

Prep Time: 10 minutes

Marinating Time: 30 minutes to 2 hours

Cook Time: 12–15 minutes

Instructions:

1. In a small mixing bowl, whisk together the olive oil, lemon zest, lemon juice, minced garlic, chopped fresh parsley, chopped fresh thyme, chopped fresh rosemary, salt, and pepper to make the lemon-herb marinade.

2. Place the chicken breasts in a shallow dish or resealable plastic bag. Pour the marinade over the chicken, making

sure they are evenly coated. Cover the dish or seal the bag and refrigerate for at least 30 minutes to marinate, or up to 2 hours for maximum flavour.

3. Preheat the grill to medium-high heat.

4. Remove the chicken breasts from the marinade and discard any excess marinade.

5. Place the chicken breasts on the preheated grill. Grill for 6-7 minutes per side, or until the chicken is cooked through and the internal temperature reaches 165°F (75°C), as measured with a meat thermometer.

6. Once done, remove the grilled chicken breasts from the grill and let them rest for a few minutes before serving.

7. Serve the grilled lemon-herb chicken breasts hot, garnished with additional chopped fresh herbs if desired.

Optional serving suggestion:

• Serve the grilled chicken breasts with a side of roasted vegetables or a fresh garden salad for a complete and nutritious meal.

Nutritional information (per serving):

• Calories: 250

• Protein: 25g

• Carbohydrates: 2g

• Fat: 15g

• Fibre: 1g

Turkey and Vegetable Meatloaf

Ingredients:

For the meatloaf:

- 1 lb. lean ground turkey
- 1 small onion, finely chopped
- 1 bell pepper, finely chopped
- 1 carrot, grated
- 2 cloves garlic, minced
- 1/2 cup rolled oats
- 1/4 cup low-sodium tomato sauce
- 1 tablespoon Worcestershire sauce (optional)
- 1 teaspoon dried thyme
- 1 teaspoon dried oregano
- 1/2 teaspoon paprika
- Salt and pepper to taste
- Cooking spray or olive oil for greasing

For the Glaze:

- 1/4 cup low-sodium tomato sauce
- 1 tablespoon of honey or maple syrup
- 1 teaspoon Dijon mustard

Servings: 4-6

Prep Time: 15 minutes

Cook Time: 45 minutes

Instructions:

1. Preheat the oven to 375°F (190°C). Lightly grease a loaf pan with cooking spray or olive oil.

2. In a large mixing bowl, combine the lean ground turkey,

finely chopped onion, finely chopped bell pepper, grated carrot, minced garlic, rolled oats, low-sodium tomato sauce, Worcestershire sauce (if using), dried thyme, dried oregano, paprika, salt, and pepper. Mix until well combined.

3. Transfer the mixture to the prepared loaf pan, pressing it down evenly to form a loaf shape.

4. In a small bowl, whisk together the low-sodium tomato sauce, honey or maple syrup, and Dijon mustard to make the glaze.

5. Spread the glaze evenly over the top of the meatloaf.

6. Bake in the preheated oven for 40–45 minutes, or until the meatloaf is cooked through and the top is golden brown.

7. Once done, remove the meatloaf from the oven and let it rest for a few minutes before slicing.

8. Slice the turkey and vegetable meatloaf into thick slices and serve hot.

9. Optionally, garnish with chopped fresh parsley before serving.

Optional serving suggestion:

• Serve the turkey and vegetable meatloaf slices with a side of steamed vegetables and mashed potatoes for a classic comfort food meal.

Nutritional Information (per serving, based on 4 servings):

• Calories: 250

• Protein: 25g

• Carbohydrates: 20g

- Fat: 8g

- Fibre: 4g

Baked Salmon with Herbed Quinoa Pilaf
Ingredients:

For the baked salmon:

- 4 salmon fillets (about 6 oz each), skin-on or skinless

- 2 tablespoons of olive oil

- 2 cloves garlic, minced

- 1 teaspoon lemon zest

- 1 tablespoon of lemon juice

- 1 teaspoon dried oregano

- 1 teaspoon dried thyme

- Salt and pepper to taste

- Lemon slices for garnish (optional)

- Chopped fresh parsley for garnish (optional)

For the Herbed Quinoa Pilaf:

- 1 cup quinoa, rinsed

- 2 cups low-sodium chicken or vegetable broth

- 1 tablespoon of olive oil

- 1 small onion, finely chopped

- 2 cloves garlic, minced

- 1 carrot, diced

- 1 zucchini, diced

- 1 teaspoon dried thyme

- 1 teaspoon dried rosemary

- Salt and pepper to taste

- Chopped fresh parsley for garnish

Servings: 4

Prep Time: 15 minutes

Cook Time: 25 minutes

Instructions:

1. Preheat the oven to 400°F (200°C). Line a baking sheet with parchment paper, or lightly grease it with olive oil.

2. In a small bowl, whisk together the olive oil, minced garlic, lemon zest, lemon juice, dried oregano, dried thyme, salt, and pepper to make the marinade for the salmon.

3. Place the salmon fillets on the prepared baking sheet. Brush the marinade over the salmon fillets, coating them evenly.

4. If desired, place a few lemon slices on top of each salmon fillet for extra flavour.

5. Bake the salmon in the preheated oven for 12–15 minutes, or until the salmon flakes easily with a fork and is cooked to your desired doneness.

6. While the salmon is baking, prepare the herbed quinoa pilaf. In a medium saucepan, heat the olive oil over medium heat.

7. Add the finely chopped onion and minced garlic to the saucepan. Sauté for 2-3 minutes until softened and fragrant.

8. Add the diced carrot and diced zucchini to the saucepan. Cook for another 3–4 minutes, stirring occasionally, until

the vegetables are slightly softened.

9. Add the rinsed quinoa to the saucepan and stir to coat it in the oil and vegetables.

10. Pour in the low-sodium chicken or vegetable broth and add the dried thyme, dried rosemary, salt, and pepper. Stir well to combine.

11. Bring the mixture to a boil, then reduce the heat to low. Cover the saucepan and simmer for 15-20 minutes, or until the quinoa is cooked and the liquid is absorbed.

12. Once done, fluff the quinoa pilaf with a fork and remove it from the heat.

13. Serve the baked salmon hot alongside the herbed quinoa pilaf.

14. Garnish with chopped fresh parsley before serving.

Optional serving suggestion:

• Serve the baked salmon with a side of steamed green beans or roasted asparagus for a complete and nutritious meal.

Nutritional information (per serving):

• Calories: 400

• Protein: 30g

• Carbohydrates: 30g

• Fat: 18g

• Fibre: 5g

CHAPTER FOUR

Healthy Fats Recipes

Smashed Chickpea Avocado Salad Sandwich

Ingredients:

For the Smashed Chickpea Avocado Salad:

• 1 (15 oz) can chickpeas, drained and rinsed

• 1 ripe avocado

• 2 tablespoons of lemon juice

• 2 tablespoons chopped fresh cilantro or parsley

• 1/4 teaspoon garlic powder

• Salt and pepper to taste

• Optional add-ins: diced red onion, diced bell pepper, cherry tomatoes, diced cucumber

For the sandwich:

• 8 slices of whole-grain bread

• Lettuce leaves

• Sliced tomato

• Sliced cucumber

• Sliced red onion (optional)

Servings: 4

Prep Time: 10 minutes

Instructions:

1. In a mixing bowl, add the drained and rinsed chickpeas. Using a fork or potato masher, gently smash the chickpeas until they are partially mashed, leaving some whole chickpeas for texture.

2. Cut the ripe avocado in half, remove the pit, and scoop the flesh into the bowl with the mashed chickpeas.

3. Add lemon juice, chopped fresh cilantro or parsley, garlic powder, salt, and pepper to the bowl.

4. Mix all the ingredients together until well combined and the avocado is evenly distributed, coating the chickpeas.

5. Taste and adjust seasoning as needed, adding more lemon juice, salt, or pepper if desired.

6. To assemble the sandwiches, lay out 4 slices of whole-grain bread on a clean surface.

7. Place lettuce leaves on each slice of bread, followed by a generous scoop of the smashed chickpea avocado salad.

8. Top the salad with sliced tomato, cucumber, and red onion (if using).

9. Place the remaining 4 slices of whole-grain bread on top to close the sandwiches.

10. Cut the sandwiches in half diagonally and serve immediately, or wrap them tightly in parchment paper or plastic wrap for later.

Optional serving suggestion:

• Serve the smashed chickpea avocado salad sandwiches with a side of carrot sticks, celery, or whole-grain tortilla chips for a complete and satisfying meal.

Nutritional information (per serving):

• Calories: 350

• Protein: 12g

• Carbohydrates: 50g

• Fat: 14g

• Fibre: 10g

Almond-crusted baked chicken tenders
Ingredients:

For the chicken tenders:

• 1 lb. boneless, skinless chicken breast tenders (about 8 tenders)

• 1 cup almond flour or almond meal

• 1/2 cup grated Parmesan cheese

• 1 teaspoon garlic powder

• 1 teaspoon smoked paprika

• 1/2 teaspoon dried thyme

• 1/2 teaspoon salt

• 1/4 teaspoon black pepper

• 2 large eggs

• Cooking spray or olive oil for greasing

For the Dipping Sauce (optional):

• 1/4 cup Greek yoghurt or mayonnaise

• 1 tablespoon Dijon mustard

- 1 tablespoon of honey or maple syrup

- 1 tablespoon of lemon juice

- Salt and pepper to taste

Servings: 4

Prep Time: 15 minutes

Cook Time: 20 minutes

Instructions:

1. Preheat the oven to 400°F (200°C). Line a baking sheet with parchment paper, or lightly grease it with cooking spray or olive oil.

2. In a shallow dish, combine the almond flour, grated Parmesan cheese, garlic powder, smoked paprika, dried thyme, salt, and black pepper. Mix well to combine.

3. In another shallow dish, beat the eggs until well mixed.

4. Dip each chicken tender into the beaten eggs, allowing any excess to drip off.

5. Then, dredge the chicken tender in the almond flour mixture, pressing gently to coat it evenly on all sides.

6. Place the coated chicken tender on the prepared baking sheet. Repeat the process with the remaining chicken tenders.

7. Lightly spray the tops of the chicken tenders with cooking spray or drizzle with a little olive oil.

8. Bake in the preheated oven for 18–20 minutes, or until the chicken is cooked through and the coating is golden brown and crispy.

9. While the chicken tenders are baking, prepare the

dipping sauce, if desired. In a small bowl, whisk together the Greek yoghurt or mayonnaise, Dijon mustard, honey or maple syrup, lemon juice, salt, and pepper until smooth and well combined.

10. Once the chicken tenders are done baking, remove them from the oven and let them cool for a few minutes.

11. Serve the almond-crusted baked chicken tenders hot with the dipping sauce on the side.

Optional serving suggestion:

• Serve the chicken tenders with a side of steamed vegetables or a fresh green salad for a complete and nutritious meal.

Nutritional information (per serving, including dipping sauce):

• Calories: 350

• Protein: 30g

• Carbohydrates: 15g

• Fat: 18g

• Fibre: 5g

Creamy Avocado Pasta with Cherry Tomatoes

Ingredients:

• 8 oz (225g) pasta of your choice (such as spaghetti, linguine, or fettuccine)

• 2 ripe avocados

• 1 cup cherry tomatoes, halved

• 2 cloves garlic, minced

• 1/4 cup fresh basil leaves, chopped

- 2 tablespoons of lemon juice

- 1/4 cup grated Parmesan cheese (optional; omit for vegan version)

- Salt and pepper to taste

- Red pepper flakes (optional, for added spice)

- Extra virgin olive oil for drizzling

Servings: 4

Prep Time: 10 minutes

Cook Time: 10 minutes

Instructions:

1. Cook the pasta according to the package instructions until al dente. Drain and set aside, reserving about 1/2 cup of pasta water.

2. While the pasta is cooking, prepare the creamy avocado sauce. Cut the avocados in half, remove the pits, and scoop the flesh into a blender or food processor.

3. Add the minced garlic, lemon juice, grated Parmesan cheese (if using), chopped basil leaves, salt, and pepper to the blender or food processor with the avocado.

4. Blend until smooth and creamy, scraping down the sides as needed. If the sauce is too thick, you can thin it out with a little bit of reserved pasta water until you reach your desired consistency.

5. In a large mixing bowl, toss the cooked pasta with the creamy avocado sauce until well coated.

6. Add the halved cherry tomatoes to the pasta and gently toss to combine.

7. Taste and adjust seasoning as needed, adding more salt, pepper, or lemon juice if desired.

8. Divide the creamy avocado pasta among serving plates or bowls.

9. Drizzle with a little extra virgin olive oil and sprinkle with red pepper flakes for added spice, if desired.

10. Serve the creamy avocado pasta immediately, garnished with additional grated Parmesan cheese and fresh basil leaves if desired.

Optional serving suggestion:

• Serve the creamy avocado pasta with a side of garlic bread or a fresh green salad for a complete and satisfying meal.

Nutritional information (per serving):

• Calories: 350

• Protein: 8g

• Carbohydrates: 45g

• Fat: 15g

• Fibre: 10g

Kale Salad with Creamy Tahini Dressing

Ingredients:

For the salad:

• 1 bunch of kale (about 8 oz.), stems removed, and leaves thinly sliced

• 1/2 cup cherry tomatoes, halved

• 1/4 cup sliced red onion

• 1/4 cup grated carrots

- 1/4 cup sliced cucumber

- 1/4 cup cooked quinoa (optional, for added protein and texture)

- 2 tablespoons toasted sunflower seeds or pumpkin seeds

- 2 tablespoons chopped fresh parsley or cilantro (optional, for garnish)

- Salt and pepper to taste

For the creamy tahini dressing:

- 1/4 cup tahini

- 2 tablespoons of lemon juice

- 2 tablespoons of water

- 1 tablespoon of maple syrup or honey

- 1 clove garlic, minced

- 1/2 teaspoon ground cumin

- Salt and pepper to taste

Servings: 4

Prep Time: 15 minutes

Instructions:

1. In a large mixing bowl, add the thinly sliced kale leaves. Drizzle with a little olive oil, and sprinkle with a pinch of salt.

2. Massage the kale leaves with your hands for 2-3 minutes, or until the leaves are tender and wilted.

3. Add the halved cherry tomatoes, sliced red onion, grated carrots, sliced cucumber, and cooked quinoa (if using) to the bowl with the massaged kale.

4. In a small bowl, whisk together all the ingredients for the creamy tahini dressing until smooth and well combined.

5. Pour the creamy tahini dressing over the kale salad ingredients in the bowl.

6. Toss gently to coat everything evenly in the dressing.

7. Season with additional salt and pepper to taste, if needed.

8. Transfer the kale salad to serving plates or bowls.

9. Sprinkle with toasted sunflower seeds or pumpkin seeds and chopped fresh parsley or cilantro for garnish.

10. Serve the kale salad immediately as a side dish or light meal.

Optional serving suggestion:

• Serve the kale salad with grilled chicken, tofu, or chickpeas for added protein, or alongside a slice of whole-grain bread for a complete and satisfying meal.

Nutritional information (per serving):

• Calories: 250

• Protein: 7g

• Carbohydrates: 20g

• Fat: 15g

• Fibre: 5g

Coconut-Curry Tofu Stir-Fry

Ingredients:

For the stir-fry:

• 14 oz (400g) firm tofu, pressed and cubed

- 2 tablespoons coconut oil or vegetable oil
- 1 small onion, thinly sliced
- 2 cloves garlic, minced
- 1 bell pepper, thinly sliced
- 1 cup of broccoli florets
- 1 carrot, julienned
- 1 cup snap peas or snow peas
- 1 can (14 oz) of coconut milk
- 2 tablespoons of red curry paste
- 1 tablespoon soy sauce or tamari
- 1 tablespoon of maple syrup or brown sugar
- Salt and pepper to taste
- Cooked rice or noodles for serving

For Garnish:

- Fresh cilantro, chopped
- Lime wedges

Servings: 4

Prep Time: 15 minutes

Cook Time: 20 minutes

Instructions:

1. Press the tofu to remove excess moisture. Once pressed, cut the tofu into cubes and set them aside.

2. In a large skillet or wok, heat the coconut oil over medium heat. Add the sliced onion and minced garlic, and sauté for 2-3 minutes until fragrant.

3. Add the cubed tofu to the skillet and cook for 5-7 minutes, stirring occasionally, until the tofu is golden brown and slightly crispy on all sides. Remove the tofu from the skillet and set it aside.

4. In the same skillet, add a little more oil, if needed. Add the sliced bell pepper, broccoli florets, julienned carrot, and snap peas or snow peas. Stir-fry for 3–4 minutes until the vegetables are crisp-tender.

5. In a small bowl, whisk together the coconut milk, red curry paste, soy sauce or tamari, and maple syrup or brown sugar until smooth.

6. Pour the coconut milk mixture into the skillet with the vegetables. Bring to a simmer and cook for 2-3 minutes, stirring occasionally, until the sauce has thickened slightly.

7. Add the cooked tofu back to the skillet and stir to coat it evenly in the sauce.

8. Season with salt and pepper to taste, adjusting the seasoning as needed.

9. Remove the skillet from the heat and serve the coconut-curry tofu stir-fry hot over cooked rice or noodles.

10. Garnish with chopped fresh cilantro and lime wedges for added flavour.

Optional serving suggestion:

• Serve the coconut-curry tofu stir-fry with a side of steamed jasmine rice or noodles, and garnish with additional sliced chilli peppers for extra heat if desired.

Nutritional information (per serving, without rice or noodles):

• Calories: 300

- Protein: 10g

- Carbohydrates: 15g

- Fat: 25g

- Fibre: 5g

Avocado and Black Bean Quesadillas

Ingredients:

- 4 large flour tortillas

- 1 ripe avocado, peeled, pitted, and sliced

- 1 cup cooked black beans, drained and rinsed

- 1 cup shredded cheddar or Monterey Jack cheese

- 1/2 cup corn kernels (fresh, canned, or frozen)

- 1/4 cup diced red onion

- 1/4 cup chopped fresh cilantro

- 1 teaspoon ground cumin

- 1 teaspoon chilli powder

- Salt and pepper to taste

- Cooking spray or vegetable oil for cooking

- Salsa, guacamole, or sour cream for serving (optional)

Servings: 4

Prep Time: 10 minutes

Cook Time: 10 minutes

Instructions:

1. In a mixing bowl, combine the cooked black beans, corn kernels, diced red onion, chopped cilantro, ground cumin, chilli powder, salt, and pepper. Mix well to combine.

2. Heat a large skillet or griddle over medium heat. Lightly spray one side of a flour tortilla with cooking spray or brush it with vegetable oil.

3. Place the tortilla, oil-side down, in the skillet. Spread a quarter of the black bean mixture evenly over half of the tortilla.

4. Arrange a few slices of avocado on top of the black bean mixture, then sprinkle with shredded cheese.

5. Fold the tortilla in half to cover the filling, creating a half-moon shape.

6. Cook the quesadilla for 2-3 minutes on each side, or until golden brown and crispy and the cheese is melted.

7. Repeat the process with the remaining tortillas and filling ingredients.

8. Once cooked, transfer the quesadillas to a cutting board and let them cool for a minute.

9. Cut each quesadilla into wedges using a sharp knife or pizza cutter.

10. Serve the avocado and black bean quesadillas hot with salsa, guacamole, or sour cream on the side for dipping, if desired.

Optional serving suggestion:

• Serve the quesadillas with a side of Mexican rice and a green salad for a complete and satisfying meal.

Nutritional information (per serving, without optional toppings):

• Calories: 350

• Protein: 15g

- Carbohydrates: 40g

- Fat: 15g

- Fibre: 8g

Almond-Crusted Salmon with Lemon-Dill Sauce

Ingredients:

For the almond-crusted salmon:

- 4 salmon fillets (6 oz each), skin-on or skinless

- 1 cup almond flour or almond meal

- 1/2 cup almond slices, finely chopped

- 2 tablespoons fresh parsley, finely chopped

- 1 teaspoon lemon zest

- 1/2 teaspoon garlic powder

- 1/2 teaspoon smoked paprika

- Salt and pepper to taste

- 2 tablespoons of olive oil

For the Lemon-Dill Sauce:

- 1/2 cup Greek yoghurt or sour cream

- 2 tablespoons fresh dill, finely chopped

- 1 tablespoon of lemon juice

- 1 teaspoon lemon zest

- Salt and pepper to taste

Servings: 4

Prep Time: 15 minutes

Cook Time: 15 minutes

Instructions:

1. Preheat the oven to 400°F (200°C). Line a baking sheet with parchment paper.

2. In a shallow dish, combine the almond flour, chopped almond slices, parsley, lemon zest, garlic powder, smoked paprika, salt, and pepper. Mix well to combine.

3. Pat the salmon fillets dry with paper towels. If using skin-on salmon, place the fillets skin-side down on the prepared baking sheet. If using skinless salmon, place the fillets directly on the baking sheet.

4. Drizzle olive oil over each salmon fillet, then spread it evenly over the surface.

5. Press each salmon fillet into the almond mixture, coating it generously on all sides and pressing gently to adhere to the almond crust.

6. Bake the almond-crusted salmon in the preheated oven for 12–15 minutes, or until the salmon is cooked through and the almond crust is golden brown and crispy.

7. While the salmon is baking, prepare the lemon-dill sauce. In a small bowl, combine the Greek yoghurt or sour cream, chopped fresh dill, lemon juice, lemon zest, salt, and pepper. Stir well to combine.

8. Once the salmon is done baking, remove it from the oven and let it rest for a few minutes.

9. Serve the almond-crusted salmon hot, topped with a dollop of lemon-dill sauce.

10. Garnish with additional chopped fresh dill and lemon slices, if desired.

Optional serving suggestion:

• Serve the almond-crusted salmon with a side of steamed vegetables or a fresh green salad for a complete and nutritious meal.

Nutritional information (per serving, including lemon-dill sauce):

• Calories: 400

• Protein: 30g

• Carbohydrates: 10g

• Fat: 25g

• Fibre: 3g

Greek Yoghurt Chicken Salad with Grapes and Walnuts
Ingredients:

• 2 cups cooked chicken breast, diced or shredded

• 1 cup seedless grapes, halved

• 1/2 cup walnuts, chopped

• 1/4 cup celery, finely chopped

• 1/4 cup red onion, finely chopped

• 1/4 cup plain Greek yoghurt

• 1 tablespoon of lemon juice

• 1 tablespoon of honey or maple syrup

• 1 tablespoon Dijon mustard

• Salt and pepper to taste

• Fresh parsley or dill for garnish (optional)

Servings: 4

Prep Time: 15 minutes

Instructions:

1. In a large mixing bowl, combine the cooked chicken breast, halved grapes, chopped walnuts, finely chopped celery, and finely chopped red onion.

2. In a small bowl, whisk together the plain Greek yoghurt, lemon juice, honey or maple syrup, Dijon mustard, salt, and pepper until smooth and well combined.

3. Pour the Greek yoghurt dressing over the chicken salad ingredients in the large mixing bowl.

4. Gently toss to coat everything evenly in the dressing.

5. Taste and adjust seasoning as needed, adding more salt, pepper, lemon juice, or honey/maple syrup to taste.

6. Once the chicken salad is well mixed and seasoned to your liking, cover and refrigerate it for at least 30 minutes to allow the flavours to meld together.

7. Before serving, garnish the Greek yoghurt chicken salad with chopped fresh parsley or dill for added flavour and freshness, if desired.

8. Serve the chicken salad chilled as a filling for sandwiches, wraps, or lettuce cups, or enjoy it on its own as a light and nutritious meal.

Optional serving suggestion:

• Serve the Greek yoghurt chicken salad on whole grain bread or lettuce leaves for a low-carb option, or alongside a green salad for a complete and satisfying meal.

Nutritional information (per serving):

• Calories: 300

• Protein: 25g

- Carbohydrates: 15g

- Fat: 15g

- Fibre: 3g

Quinoa-stuffed avocados

Ingredients:

- 2 ripe avocados

- 1 cup of cooked quinoa

- 1/2 cup black beans, drained and rinsed

- 1/2 cup corn kernels (fresh, canned, or frozen)

- 1/4 cup diced red bell pepper

- 1/4 cup diced red onion

- 1/4 cup chopped fresh cilantro

- 2 tablespoons of lime juice

- 1 tablespoon of olive oil

- 1 teaspoon ground cumin

- 1/2 teaspoon chilli powder

- Salt and pepper to taste

- Optional toppings: diced tomatoes, sliced jalapeños, shredded cheese, avocado slices, sour cream, salsa

Servings: 4

Prep Time: 15 minutes

Instructions:

1. Cut the avocados in half lengthwise and remove the pits. Scoop out a little bit of flesh from each avocado half to create a larger cavity for the filling. Set aside.

2. In a large mixing bowl, combine the cooked quinoa, black beans, corn kernels, diced red bell pepper, diced red onion, and chopped fresh cilantro.

3. In a small bowl, whisk together the lime juice, olive oil, ground cumin, chilli powder, salt, and pepper to make the dressing.

4. Pour the dressing over the quinoa mixture in the large mixing bowl.

5. Toss gently to coat everything evenly in the dressing.

6. Taste and adjust seasoning as needed, adding more salt, pepper, or lime juice if desired.

7. Spoon the quinoa mixture into the cavities of the halved avocados, dividing it evenly among them.

8. Garnish the stuffed avocados with additional chopped cilantro, diced tomatoes, sliced jalapeños, shredded cheese, avocado slices, sour cream, or salsa, if desired.

9. Serve the quinoa-stuffed avocados immediately as a nutritious and delicious appetiser, side dish, or light meal.

Optional serving suggestion:

• Serve the stuffed avocados with a side of tortilla chips or a fresh green salad for a complete and satisfying meal.

Nutritional information (per serving, based on filling only):

• Calories: 250

• Protein: 8g

• Carbohydrates: 30g

• Fat: 12g

• Fibre: 8g

Almond and Apricot Energy Bites

Ingredients:

• 1 cup rolled oats

• 1/2 cup almond butter

• 1/4 cup honey or maple syrup

• 1/4 cup chopped almonds

• 1/4 cup chopped dried apricots

• 2 tablespoons ground flaxseed or chia seeds

• 1/2 teaspoon vanilla extract

• Pinch of salt

• Optional: shredded coconut, cocoa powder, or additional chopped nuts for coating.

Servings: Makes about 12–16 energy bites.

Prep Time: 15 minutes

Instructions:

1. In a large mixing bowl, combine the rolled oats, almond butter, honey or maple syrup, chopped almonds, chopped dried apricots, ground flaxseed or chia seeds, vanilla extract, and a pinch of salt.

2. Stir the mixture until well combined and sticky. If the mixture seems too dry, you can add a little more almond butter or honey or maple syrup to help bind everything together.

3. Once the mixture is well combined, cover the bowl and refrigerate it for at least 30 minutes to allow it to firm up slightly, which will make it easier to roll into balls.

4. After chilling, remove the mixture from the refrigerator. Using clean hands, scoop out a small portion of the mixture and roll it between your palms to form a ball about 1 inch in diameter.

5. Continue rolling the mixture into balls until you've used up all the mixture.

6. Optional: Roll the energy bites in shredded coconut, cocoa powder, or additional chopped nuts for extra flavour and texture.

7. Once all the energy bites are rolled, transfer them to an airtight container and store them in the refrigerator for up to one week.

8. Enjoy the almond and apricot energy bites as a nutritious and delicious snack whenever you need a quick boost of energy!

Optional serving suggestion:

• Serve the energy bites with a glass of almond milk or your favourite yoghurt for a satisfying and nourishing snack.

Nutritional information (per energy bite):

• Calories: 100

• Protein: 3g

• Carbohydrates: 12g

• Fat: 5g

• Fibre: 2g

Spicy Avocado Chickpea Salad

Ingredients:

• 1 can (15 oz) chickpeas, drained and rinsed

- 1 ripe avocado, peeled, pitted, and diced
- 1/4 cup diced red onion
- 1/4 cup chopped fresh cilantro
- 1 jalapeño pepper, seeded and finely diced
- 1 tablespoon of lime juice
- 1 tablespoon of olive oil
- 1/2 teaspoon ground cumin
- 1/4 teaspoon chilli powder
- Salt and pepper to taste

Servings: 2-4

Prep Time: 10 minutes

Instructions:

1. In a large mixing bowl, combine the drained and rinsed chickpeas, diced avocado, diced red onion, chopped fresh cilantro, and finely diced jalapeño pepper.

2. In a small bowl, whisk together the lime juice, olive oil, ground cumin, chilli powder, salt, and pepper to make the dressing.

3. Pour the dressing over the chickpea mixture in the large mixing bowl.

4. Gently toss to coat everything evenly in the dressing.

5. Taste and adjust seasoning as needed, adding more salt, pepper, lime juice, or chilli powder if desired.

6. Once the salad is well mixed and seasoned to your liking, cover and refrigerate it for at least 30 minutes to allow the flavours to meld together.

7. Before serving, give the spicy avocado chickpea salad a final toss and adjust seasoning if needed.

8. Serve the salad chilled as a refreshing and flavorful side dish or light meal.

Optional serving suggestion:

• Serve the spicy avocado chickpea salad on a bed of mixed greens or baby spinach for added freshness, or as a filling for tacos, wraps, or sandwiches.

Nutritional Information (per serving, based on 4 servings):

• Calories: 180

• Protein: 6g

• Carbohydrates: 18g

• Fat: 10g

• Fibre: 7g

Chia Seed Pudding with Berries

Ingredients:

• 1/4 cup chia seeds

• 1 cup unsweetened almond milk or any milk of your choice

• 1 tablespoon honey or maple syrup (optional)

• 1/2 teaspoon vanilla extract

• 1/2 cup mixed berries (such as strawberries, blueberries, or raspberries)

• Fresh mint leaves for garnish (optional)

Servings: 2

Prep Time: 5 minutes

Chilling Time: 2 hours or overnight

Instructions:

1. In a mixing bowl or jar, combine the chia seeds, almond milk, honey or maple syrup (if using), and vanilla extract. Stir well to combine.

2. Cover the bowl or jar and refrigerate the chia seed mixture for at least 2 hours, or preferably overnight, to allow it to thicken and set into a pudding-like consistency.

3. After the chilling time, remove the chia seed pudding from the refrigerator and give it a good stir to redistribute the seeds.

4. Divide the chia seed pudding into serving bowls or glasses.

5. Top each serving of chia seed pudding with a generous portion of mixed berries.

6. Garnish with fresh mint leaves, if desired, for a pop of colour and extra freshness.

7. Serve the chia seed pudding with berries immediately as a nutritious and delicious breakfast, snack, or dessert.

Optional serving suggestions:

• Drizzle the chia seed pudding with a little extra honey or maple syrup for added sweetness, if desired.

• Serve the pudding with a dollop of Greek yoghurt or coconut yoghurt for extra creaminess and protein.

• Sprinkle with a handful of granola or chopped nuts for added texture and crunch.

Nutritional information (per serving):

• Calories: 150

- Protein: 4g

- Carbohydrates: 20g

- Fat: 7g

- Fibre: 10g

Mediterranean Chickpea Salad with Olive Oil Dressing

Ingredients:

For the salad:

- 2 cans (15 oz each) chickpeas, drained and rinsed

- 1 English cucumber, diced

- 1 cup cherry tomatoes, halved

- 1/2 cup Kalamata olives, pitted and halved

- 1/4 cup red onion, thinly sliced

- 1/4 cup fresh parsley, chopped

- 1/4 cup fresh mint leaves, chopped

- 1/4 cup crumbled feta cheese (optional)

For the dressing:

- 1/4 cup extra-virgin olive oil

- 2 tablespoons of red wine vinegar

- 1 tablespoon of lemon juice

- 1 clove garlic, minced

- 1 teaspoon dried oregano

- Salt and pepper to taste

Servings: 4-6

Prep Time: 15 minutes

Instructions:

1. In a large mixing bowl, combine the drained and rinsed chickpeas, diced cucumber, halved cherry tomatoes, halved Kalamata olives, thinly sliced red onion, chopped fresh parsley, and chopped fresh mint leaves.

2. In a small bowl, whisk together the extra virgin olive oil, red wine vinegar, lemon juice, minced garlic, dried oregano, salt, and pepper to make the dressing.

3. Pour the dressing over the chickpea salad in the large mixing bowl.

4. Gently toss to coat everything evenly in the dressing.

5. Taste and adjust seasoning as needed, adding more salt, pepper, or lemon juice if desired.

6. If using, sprinkle the crumbled feta cheese over the salad and toss lightly to incorporate.

7. Once the salad is well mixed and seasoned to your liking, cover and refrigerate it for at least 30 minutes to allow the flavours to meld together.

8. Before serving, give the Mediterranean chickpea salad a final toss and adjust seasoning if needed.

9. Serve the salad chilled as a refreshing and flavorful side dish or light meal.

Optional serving suggestion:

• Serve the Mediterranean chickpea salad with grilled chicken, fish, or lamb for a complete and satisfying meal.

Nutritional Information (per serving, based on 4 servings without feta cheese):

• Calories: 300

- Protein: 10g

- Carbohydrates: 30g

- Fat: 15g

- Fibre: 8g

Avocado and White Bean Wrap

Ingredients:

- 1 ripe avocado, peeled, pitted, and sliced

- 1 can (15 oz) white beans, drained and rinsed

- 1/4 cup diced red onion

- 1/4 cup diced red bell pepper

- 1/4 cup chopped fresh cilantro

- 1 tablespoon of lime juice

- 1 tablespoon of olive oil

- 1/2 teaspoon ground cumin

- Salt and pepper to taste

- 4 whole wheat or spinach tortillas

- Optional: shredded lettuce, sliced tomatoes, grated cheese, and hot sauce

Servings: 4

Prep Time: 15 minutes

Instructions:

1. In a mixing bowl, combine the drained and rinsed white beans, diced red onion, diced red bell pepper, chopped fresh cilantro, lime juice, olive oil, ground cumin, salt, and pepper. Mash the mixture slightly with a fork or potato masher until it reaches a chunky consistency.

2. Lay out the tortillas on a clean work surface.

3. Divide the mashed white bean mixture evenly among the tortillas, spreading it out in a line down the centre of each tortilla.

4. Top the white bean mixture on each tortilla with slices of ripe avocado.

5. Optional: Add shredded lettuce, sliced tomatoes, grated cheese, or hot sauce on top of the avocado layer for extra flavour and texture.

6. Fold the sides of each tortilla inward, then roll up tightly from the bottom to enclose the filling and form a wrap.

7. Serve the avocado and white bean wraps immediately, or wrap them tightly in foil or parchment paper for easy transport.

8. Enjoy the wraps as a nutritious and satisfying lunch, dinner, or on-the-go meal option.

Optional serving suggestion:

• Serve the wraps with a side of salsa, Greek yoghurt, or guacamole for dipping, or alongside a green salad for a complete and balanced meal.

Nutritional information (per serving):

• Calories: 300

• Protein: 9g

• Carbohydrates: 38g

• Fat: 13g

• Fibre: 8g

Almond Butter Banana Smoothie

Ingredients:

• 2 ripe bananas, peeled and sliced

• 2 tablespoons of almond butter

• 1 cup unsweetened almond milk or any milk of your choice

• 1/2 cup plain Greek yoghurt or dairy-free yoghurt

• 1 tablespoon honey or maple syrup (optional)

• 1/2 teaspoon vanilla extract

• 1/4 teaspoon ground cinnamon

• 4-6 ice cubes

Servings: 2

Prep Time: 5 minutes

Instructions:

1. In a blender, combine the sliced bananas, almond butter, almond milk, Greek yoghurt, honey or maple syrup (if using), vanilla extract, ground cinnamon, and ice cubes.

2. Blend on high speed until the ingredients are smooth and creamy and the ice cubes are completely crushed.

3. Taste the smoothie and adjust sweetness or thickness by adding more honey or maple syrup, if desired, or more almond milk if you prefer a thinner consistency.

4. Once the desired consistency and sweetness are achieved, blend again briefly to combine.

5. Pour the almond butter banana smoothie into glasses and serve immediately.

Optional serving suggestion:

· Garnish the smoothie with a sprinkle of ground cinnamon or a drizzle of almond butter for added flavour and presentation.

Nutritional information (per serving):

· Calories: 250

· Protein: 8g

· Carbohydrates: 30g

· Fat: 12g

· Fibre: 5g

CONCLUSION

In closing, the Ornish diet isn't just a prescription for physical health; it's a holistic blueprint for living with vitality, purpose, and joy. By nourishing your body with vibrant plant-based foods, moving with intention, taming stress, and fostering meaningful connections, you're not just transforming your health—you're embracing a lifestyle of empowerment and resilience.

As you embark on this journey, remember that change is not about perfection but about progress. Each step you take towards prioritising your health is a testament to your commitment to self-care and well-being. So savour each bite, move with grace, and embrace the journey with an open heart.

Together, let's rewrite the narrative of health and vitality. Here's to a future filled with boundless energy, radiant health, and the joy of living well. Welcome to the Ornish lifestyle—a journey of transformation, one mindful choice at a time.